the long way **home** Marian Ritchie

A Journey Through Alzheimer's

HARROP PRESS

Ontario, Canada

THE LONG WAY HOME
Copyright © 2005, Marian Ritchie

All Scripture quotations, unless otherwise specified, are from *The Holy Bible, King James Version.* Copyright © 1977, 1984, Thomas Nelson Inc., Publishers.

ISBN: 0-9737682-0-7
Previously published by Essence Publishing under ISBN 1-55306-683-9

Library and Archives Canada Cataloguing in Publication
Ritchie, Marian, 1940-
    The long way home : a journey through Alzheimer's / Marian Ritchie.
ISBN 0-9737682-0-7
    1. Smith, Edwin--Health. 2. Alzheimer's disease--Patients--Canada--Biography. 3. Alzheimer's disease--Popular works. I. Title.
RC523.2.R58 2005   362.196'831'0092   C2005-902456-9

For more information or
to order additional copies, please contact:

Marian Ritchie
E-mail: marianritchie@sympatico.ca

Harrop Press
30 Harrop Avenue
Georgetown, ON L7G 5R4, Canada

Tel: (905) 702-9364 • Fax: (905) 702-8158

Printed in Canada

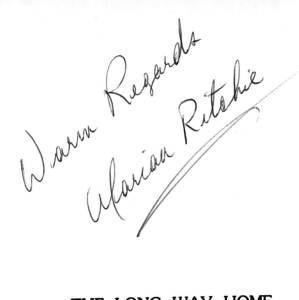

Warm Regards
Marian Ritchie

THE LONG WAY HOME

A Journey Through Alzheimer's

*This book is dedicated
in loving memory
of Edwin*

Table of Contents

1. The End 17

This chapter describes the dramatic onset of the disease, en-route to Florida for the winter, and its subsequent affect on every aspect of our lives, as it marked the end of everything; forcing us to start down a new and uncertain road to an unknown future.

2. Don't Let the Sun Set! 33

Here we learn more about Alzheimer's disease, including the cause of my husband's increased agitation, concurrent with the onset of evening and the setting of the sun.

3. The Third Man Theme 53

Still in Florida, we discover the existence, and later the true identity, of the mysterious third man living with us.

4. In Retrospect. 73

Back home in Canada again, we have Edwin tested and properly diagnosed. In retrospect we try to see some of the symptoms leading up to the final onset of the disease.

This is a copy of the poem I wrote for my husband's funeral, the writing of which also helped me in the process of healing, serving as a catharsis for my grief.

Preface

This book is dedicated with love and affection to a wonderful man, my late husband, Edwin, who unwittingly became the protagonist of this tragic tale, a true account of his struggle—and mine—with Alzheimer's disease. It is a story that continues to be repeated, countless times over, in millions of homes across our country and, indeed, throughout the world.

It is a somewhat poignant and penetrating account of our journey through Alzheimer's, but for the most part, it is a humorous compilation of stories and anecdotes, depicting the progression of the disease as we lived with it from day to day. If it seems disjointed and eclectic in places, it probably is, for that is what life was like for us during those years. However, I have related these events exactly as they happened, in the hope that others travelling that same road might learn to laugh in the face of fear. Laughter is after all the best medicine, and a way of preserving our sanity, so if we can learn to laugh at ourselves, and our situation, we are already halfway there.

In my heart I felt compelled to write this book, for I had a burden to share our story with the rest of the world, in the hopes that others, who are travelling even now on that same, long, dark journey, may come to realize they are not alone! Others have gone before, and still more will follow. It is inevitable! It is also inexorable, but there is hope for the future. Hang in there! Hold on, for there is light at the end of the tunnel, and you are not alone in traversing that long way home!

Acknowledgments

I wish to acknowledge those friends, acquaintances and colleagues—not necessarily mutually exclusive, one from the other—who have helped and encouraged me along my journey, and without whom, I would not have survived to write this book. I couldn't begin to mention everyone who has touched my life along the way, but I am still thankful for each one of you. If your name does not appear, please know that I am grateful nonetheless for your contribution.

MELISSA KLASSEN and CYNTHIA LEES, my loving daughters, who faithfully prayed for me, and encouraged me to follow the burden of my heart in endeavouring to write this book.

ALMA FATTORI, a true friend and a gracious lady, who has been a bulwark for me, a tower of strength, a listening ear, and a shoulder on which to cry.

PAT AND BILL WADDELL, who proved their true friendship by their actions, even more than words, and for whom I shall always be grateful.

The ALZHEIMER'S SUPPORT GROUP AT BENDALE ACRES, where I found the encouragement and support to carry on, and for the leaders of that group who sacrificed their time and energy to help those in need. KAREN NEESON and her husband, AL STRACHAN, who rescued me from the extra pressure of a recalcitrant computer, and LINDA ENGEL who helped Karen in leading the group.

SYLVIA HENSEL, from Bendale acres, a very special lady, who was instrumental in helping and encouraging me when I might have given up. She has now been promoted to glory herself, but her spirit lives on in the hearts of those she's helped along the way.

REV. CECIL WALKER, a wonderful man who was of great encouragement to our group and a true example of Christian love in action. A retired Anglican Minister, now also promoted to glory, he lovingly nursed his own wife through many years of suffering with Alzheimer's, while helping others in similar situations.

MIA KING, a very special friend who shared her strength and wisdom with me, and JEAN WULKAN, another good friend, who also bore the burden of having her husband in a nursing home. I will always be grateful for the love they showed me and the special blend of "harmony" they both contributed, helping to make music out of the jumbled cacophony my life had become during some exceedingly dark days.

JEAN MAASKANT, a dear friend and fellow traveller on her own journey with Alzheimer's, lovingly caring for her husband in his struggle with the dreaded disease.

LEISUREWORLD NURSING HOME and all who labour there, from the Director of the Home, and the Doctors who care for the patients, to the Activation Department, the volunteers, and even the housekeeping staff, all of whom contributed in no small way to the care, comfort and well-being of my husband during his years at the nursing home. I could not have asked for better care and I am grateful to them all. A special thank-you to LUNA and ANNIE in Activation, along with ANDREW GOSS, head of the Activation Department.

A very special word of thanks to the Nurses and Nursing Assistants, who lovingly laboured on the Alzheimer's ward at Leisureworld. In particular I am grateful to JANET, GEMA, SANDI, and MIKE, whose caring attitudes added greatly to my husband's quality of life.

RICHARD CLAYTON and the staff at the TRULL FUNERAL HOME, who went above and beyond the call of duty in helping me through some very difficult days.

Last but not least, to the wonderful people at EGLINTON ST. GEORGES, and all my friends and co-workers, who stood with me and encouraged me along the way, giving me the confidence of knowing I was not alone in my struggle. They had a special way of letting me know they were there for me, and I shall always appreciate them and the Christian love they showed.

The End

CHAPTER 1

"Where am I?"
"What's happening?"
"Why am I so cold?"

These plaintive cries rent the night air, piercing through the fog of sleep as I struggled to emerge from its tenuous grasp. The darkness was complete, as not even a glimmer of light managed to penetrate the curtains on the far wall of the room and I floundered helplessly, trying to find the light switch, wanting to dispel the darkness and, hopefully, the feeling of panic that rose in my breast, as the frightening cries continued to assault the blackness of the night. At last, my fumbling fingers found the lamp by the bedside and managed to locate the switch, but the sudden transformation was too painful for my sleep-laden eyes and I was forced to squeeze them tightly shut again until they could adjust to the light. It was probably only minutes, but it seemed like a long time had elapsed since my rude awakening and my subsequent realization of the problem at hand. Actually, I hoped I was still dreaming, (please God make it so), instead of facing this waking nightmare, which was in truth, only the beginning of a living nightmare of pain and suffering and unmitigated torture and humiliation. Little did I realize then that this night would spell the end of my life as I knew it, the end of peace and comfort, the end of stability, and the end of an era.

As my eyes adjusted to the light, I saw my husband standing in the middle of the room, totally naked and crying out in his distress and confusion. Desperately I tried to calm him down and quiet his wailing, but it took a long time before I was able to get through to him at all, to be able to communicate with him on any level. Even then, however, he could not relax, and continued to be extremely agitated as he was totally disorientated and terrified, not knowing where he was or why he was there.

Talking calmly and slowly, I tried again to explain to him that we were in a motel on our way to Florida, but he was still unable to grasp the import of my words. He just could not understand why we were going to Florida in the first place.

"What is Florida anyway, and why aren't we in our own home?"

"What happened to my house?"

Then, suddenly affecting an entirely different approach, he maintained that surely he must have been abducted. Perhaps someone was plotting against him and trying to steal his house. Again, just as rapidly, his thoughts were diverted in another direction and he became convinced that he had been put into jail.

The questions, and his equally inane answers, just kept coming and after a while I was at a loss as to how to answer him, as his confused mind vividly explored all these varied scenarios. My explanations to his deluge of questions were repeatedly refused, and he continued to ask them over and over until I almost became desperate myself.

As the questioning continued, his manner grew more and more aggressive, ranging from fear, to anger, and then to hostility, until I feared the outcome.

"Have we been arrested?" he yelled.

"Are we in jail?"

"Why are we here?"

"Have we been in an accident?"

I kept trying to reassure him, telling him that everything was all right and not to worry. Then he'd counter with more questions.

"How do you know we're all right?"

"It's O.K. love," I'd try again, "We're in a motel on our way to Florida."

"Florida!" he'd scream, "Florida! Why are we going there? Anyway, how do you know these things if I don't?"

And so it would go—on and on and on!

Then I thought of another possible complication and I almost held my breath as I waited for his answer to the question that was paramount in my mind.

I said to him, "Honey, do you know who I am?"

It was a great relief to hear him say, "You're my wife, of course."

However, just as I was breathing a sigh of relief, I thought of something else and I asked him if he knew my name. He couldn't answer! He couldn't remember my name! My heart sank as I suddenly realized with painful certainty that this was no temporary anomaly. Still, with true human frailty, my heart refused to accept what my brain had already grasped, and I continued to convince myself that if only I could get him back to bed and to sleep, he'd be better in the morning. Surely this was just a nightmare, wasn't it? How could it possibly be anything else?

Again he demanded an answer to his original question, "Why is it so cold?"

"Because you insisted that I turn off the heat when we went to bed," I replied, trying to explain. "The radiator was too noisy and you couldn't sleep."

"But it's freezing bloody cold in here," he shouted, ignoring my answer.

"Well it's no wonder," I countered, as calmly as I could. "Who wouldn't be cold, standing there stark naked? Please honey, let me help you get your pyjamas on, at least. Then you'll feel better."

At last, practicality prevailed, and I managed to divert his focus from the situation to his immediate needs, slowly but surely encouraging him to don his pyjamas and crawl back into the warm bed; a task finally accomplished but not without great difficulty and much resistance on his part.

For a long time I just held him in my arms, gently stroking his brow and crooning softly, quietly saying everything I could think of, yet saying nothing at all; just sounds, comforting, soothing sounds, until at last he drifted off to sleep. I didn't turn off the light; I didn't dare to face the darkness again—not that night—maybe never!

Sleep eluded me for the remainder of the night and I did a lot of thinking, while carefully monitoring my husband's breathing, as he slept peacefully in my arms. Here we were on our way to Florida for the winter, somewhere on the other side of Cincinnati—I had no idea where—at a motel in a strange town, in another country, where we didn't know anyone, or where we were exactly. It was terrifying for me as well! Who would you call in a situation such as this? Where could one go for help? I really didn't know what to do! What could I do?

During that long night I decided that the most important thing was to get to Florida, as quickly as possible. To accomplish this we needed to drive as far as we possibly could the next day. We were too far out to return to Canada, and besides, I knew how much Edwin had been looking forward to going to Florida and escaping the cold winter back home. I couldn't deny him that! If we could just get to Florida and get settled into our condo there, I was sure that things would improve. Once my husband was able to achieve a comfortable schedule again, surely everything would be all right. (As it was, however, the "best laid plans" don't always work out and this was no exception. He didn't get better and during the following months, I agonized over what to do for him.)

The following day we got up early and dressed for breakfast. Edwin seemed to have no recollection of what had taken place during the night so I didn't remind him, other than to ask him a couple of questions. Although he was still unable to remember my name, he did recognize the hug I gave him as being familiar, so I let it go at that.

In the restaurant at breakfast, he casually asked me, "What happened to the hotel we went to last night?"

He was unable to grasp the fact that we were still in the same one and I didn't pursue the issue. He ate a good breakfast though, and seemed to be in better spirits, so I was considerably relieved. That night when we stopped at the next motel he complained loudly at dinner and ate very little. However, there was no repeat of the previous night's activities, and again I was grateful. In fact, the next morning he seemed much improved, having slept well, and was even able to joke with me about not remembering my name.

We arrived at our condo around 5:30 that evening and I got busy unloading the car. By then Edwin was disorientated again and convinced that Ontario was just down the street from where we were. In fact, he couldn't understand why we couldn't go home or even why we came to be where we were at all. He asked me what I had done with all his belongings; what about his money; who would pay his bills, etc. Then, as the evening wore on, he grew worse and worse. He soon became convinced again that he was the victim of a plot cooked up to get him away so that his son could steal all his things, (something that his son would never think of doing, I know).

Thinking to reassure him, I explained that we ourselves had made all the arrangements to come to Florida and that his son had nothing to do with it. I also mentioned how excited he had been about coming down and how he had been looking forward to it for months.

"So you see," I reiterated, "your son had nothing to do with our going to Florida. We decided on our own to come down and just told him when we were going."

Suddenly Edwin became very angry; furious with me now, because I had told him where we were going.

"Why did you have to tell him where we were?" he demanded, "It's none of his business!"

Now more than ever convinced that his son was after his money and belongings, he then accused me of being in collusion with him. He wanted to know how I had managed to drag him off to Florida. Had I drugged him and carried him out there or what? I still tried to explain that we had planned it together and that he himself had signed all the cheques for the condo. His reply was that he couldn't have signed anything when he didn't know anything about it! Thus another entire evening was spent rehashing the same conversation, with slight variations, over and over again. Everything said or even mentioned was twisted around and incorporated into his paranoia, becoming a jumbled version of nonsense.

The next day was frustratingly repetitious of the day before, and then some. Almost every ten minutes he would ask where his purse or camera bag had been hidden, convinced, of course, that someone had stolen them. I would show him where to find whatever he was looking for, and after rummaging through it, quite happily, making sure everything was still there, he would be fine—for about ten minutes or so. Then he would start all over again! As well as constantly searching for things, he would also have sporadic bouts of accusing me of putting something in his drinks, so I finally let him pour his own. Then he'd accuse me of having cooked something up with the owner of the condo. He even went so far as to ask me how long I'd been staying there before he came—as though he hadn't traveled down here with me.

Along with settling in and picking up groceries on our first full day there in Florida, we were also required to register at the office of the condo complex. I took Edwin with me of course, not daring to leave him alone, but somewhat nervous as to how he'd behave in public. I needn't have worried though, for he was as good as gold. In fact, he seemed almost normal and I was relieved, albeit quite surprised. As soon as we returned to the condo, however, he resumed his abnormal behaviour patterns: confused, questioning, and accusing, leaving me quite baffled as to what was going on in his mind.

For his birthday I gave my husband a fancy new pen to put in his shirt pocket, since he always liked to carry a pen with him. He really liked it and thanked me very much as he sat there, turning the pen over and over in his hands, admiring its shine and stroking it with his fingers. Then, suddenly, he handed the pen back to me saying, "I believe this is yours." Surprised, I returned it to him again, explaining that it was a birthday gift for him to keep in his pocket. Smiling happily, he thanked me for it, admiring it for a while as before and then, once again he turned to me, handing me the pen. Then he repeated the same words, as before, "I believe this is yours." This exchange was repeated several times until I finally put the pen in his pocket myself!

The episode of the new pen was just one of many strange interactions that occurred with my husband during those early days in Florida, and I began to realize the magnitude of what we were facing. Even his dressing took on a different fashion from his usual flair as I noticed more and more anomalies in his attire. At times he'd come out of his room wearing a clean shirt, instead of the one he'd been wearing earlier, only to re-appear a short time later, wearing another shirt on top of the first one. I'd usually ask him if he was cold and he'd say no, so I would just let him be. Extra washing I could handle. No problem! It was a lot better than arguing. It was just the strangeness of it all that baffled me, as I still didn't understand completely, what was going on in that head of his.

Every morning I'd give Edwin his blood pressure pills but one day when I gave them to him he became annoyed and said, "Is that all I get?" From then on I made sure I never left any of his pills lying around in case he decided to help himself. That was just one more thing to worry about!

One day I was taking Edwin out for a walk but he refused to leave the house because he couldn't find his RAF pin. It was in his display case back home in Canada, as he hadn't worn it for years; in fact, not since his days in the Royal Air Force. For whatever reason, that particular day he was upset, thinking somehow that he needed to be wearing his pin. I assured him repeatedly that he didn't need it and we finally started off. However, once again he balked.

"How can we go?" he demanded to know, stopping dead in his tracks. "I haven't received my flying instructions yet!" It was then I realized that he was obviously transported in time to his years in the Air Force during the war. In fact, in the days to come, he seemed to dwell more and more on his days in India, during his service with the RAF.

At times he'd have periods of lucidity, when we could converse logically, and it was during one of those times that he admitted his inability to read the newspaper any more because it was too confusing. Nothing made sense to him. I explained to him that it was part of the Alzheimer's disease and said not to worry about it, and strangely enough, he was quite content with that explanation. In fact, he even seemed pleased that there was actually a specific name for his condition. Of course, he hadn't been properly diagnosed as yet, but by that time there was little doubt in my mind as to what was his problem. Until we returned to Canada, however, we would just have to wait to have it confirmed by the doctors there. I liked those times when

Edwin could understand what I was saying to him and we could discuss his condition, along with other subjects of interest to him. I just wished he could have remembered them later. As it was, that same day he became confused again and confessed that he had no idea where he was. Poor Edwin, it must have been so bewildering for him and terribly frightening.

Chinese food was a great favourite of Edwin's and he would often ask for it, so one day I decided to treat him to supper in a Chinese restaurant. I chose one with a very good reputation so it would be special for him. The food was excellent, very fresh and tastefully prepared, and I enjoyed it thoroughly. We ordered far too much of course (doesn't everyone), so ended up eating it for the next two days. However, poor Edwin did nothing but complain throughout the meal at the restaurant and I despaired of pleasing him. Sometimes I'd wonder why I bothered trying at all. He continually complained that the food had no taste, no matter what he ate, so I finally handed him the soy sauce, telling him to add his own taste. That only made him mad, so I dropped it (not the soy sauce, just the issue!). He maintained that the restaurant should have flavoured the food properly and that he shouldn't have to add anything to make it palatable.

After returning home that evening, Edwin suddenly turned to me with an apparent thought that just occurred to him.

"Now I know what was missing at dinner!" he exclaimed. "Soy sauce! That's what we needed to add taste to the meal!"

Astounding, wasn't it? What more could I say?

Incidentally, I served the same food the next two days—with the addition of soy sauce of course—and he loved it. In fact, he was convinced that my cooking was better than the restaurant, even though I tried to explain that it was the same food.

In retrospect I do believe Edwin was actually beginning to lose his sense of taste at that point. Perhaps the disease had already started to affect that area of his brain which controls the taste buds. At any rate, I noticed a regression in his enjoyment of mealtimes. He used to derive such pleasure from good food, and fancied himself somewhat of an epicurean, so it was doubly sad for him. What a waste!

After dinner that same evening we watched a movie on television, followed by about fifteen minutes of news, during which Edwin dozed. When he awoke, I asked him if he wanted to go to bed. He said he didn't want to go alone so I promised to go with him.

"Since you watched the movie with me," I said, "I'll go to bed with you now."

"What movie?" he exclaimed. "I never watched any movie!"

"Fine," I replied, not wanting an argument, "But we can still go to bed now if you'd like."

Then he said, somewhat sullenly, "Might as well, since I'm not going to get any dinner tonight!"

I couldn't believe what I was hearing! I told him that we'd gone out to a lovely Chinese restaurant for dinner that evening but it fell on deaf ears. He wouldn't believe me! Not only could he not recall things from one day to the next, it seemed that now it applied to one hour to the next as well. It was all very distressing and bewildering, to say the least.

After settling down in Florida, I joined a local library and looked up every book I was able to find on the subject of dementia and Alzheimer's disease, already fairly certain that this was what I was facing. The books were immensely helpful and I learned a great deal, but on the other hand, the more I read, the more I became convinced that my husband really was suffering from Alzheimer's disease, and the more upset I became.

"Why me?" I cried, "And why Edwin? Why does it have to happen to us?" I agonized over these questions, calling out to God in prayer and frustration, but there was no answer!

I prayed and I cried! I even yelled at God in anger and desperation. Afterwards I'd ask God to forgive me, horrified at what I'd done—and full of remorse—but then I'd yell at him again. It just wasn't fair! We were so happy together. Why did this have to happen now—to us?

"God, why? Why are you doing this to me? Am I such a terrible person that you are punishing me? Why? Why? Why?"

Why indeed? There were no answers—I guess there never are—but I still had all those pent-up emotions and feelings to work through, and I felt so alone. Somehow *I felt like I was the only person in the whole world who had to go through what I was experiencing* and the weight of responsibility was almost unbearable.

I had always liked being a woman and having a man to do things for me, shouldering the responsibilities of life as it were. (Emancipation? Not me!) Now in one moment, one blink of the eye, my whole world had turned upside down! Everything had changed! I no longer had anyone to lean on. I had to be the strong one. I had to make the decisions, do all the driving, make all the plans—and make all the mistakes! The burden was overwhelming, and my whole existence seemed threatened. Surely I wasn't strong enough to shoulder such a great responsibility. What if I failed? What would happen to Edwin then? Thus I struggled, but ultimately I knew I had to be there for him. There was no one else and somehow I had to find the strength to go on. I had to be strong for him. He needed me and I couldn't fail him now.

And so we carried on, days and nights becoming as one, in our constant struggle to survive this terrible thing that had come to pass. Feeling alone, so very alone, and vulnerable there, in a strange place, in a strange country, away from everything and everyone I knew and trusted, yet unable to grasp completely the extent of the calamity that had befallen us. Beneath the surface, struggling for the light, was that one faint ray of hope that I refused to relinquish throughout all those long, dark days. If we could only survive the winter there, then everything would get better, especially once we returned home to our own house, in our own country, with our own friends.

It had to get better, didn't it? It couldn't be any worse!

How could I have known, that fateful night on the way to Florida, that I was facing the end: the end of life as we had known it, the end of our happiness, the end of the road. Everything was changed! Everything was different! Edwin had become someone else—a stranger to me—and I was now being forced to start down a new road, an uncertain road, and a treacherous road, to an unknown and frightening future. It was truly the end—for me—as well as for him!

Don't Let
the Sun Set!

CHAPTER 2

The days and nights that followed became a blur, as anxiety and sleeplessness robbed me of my joy and exuberance; but somehow I managed to carry on, continuing to study this terrifying disease and learning methods of coping. We found an Alzheimer's support group at the local hospital, and since I could not leave my husband alone, I took him with me. He was fully aware that something was happening to him, something called Alzheimer's disease, and was actually helpful with input in the meetings, since he still had many of his faculties at that time, especially during the daytime hours (Evenings were another story altogether!). The others in the group also appreciated his feedback and had many questions to ask him, in relation to his outlook or perspective on various aspects of the disease, and his perception of it. I also questioned the doctor about the advisability of returning home to Canada before he became any worse, but he recommended our staying for the duration of the winter, as the weather in Florida was more comfortable for my husband and he hated the cold anyway. It didn't take much persuasion as I really dreaded the thought of driving home again with Edwin in this state. The trip down had been such a nightmare that I was afraid to repeat it any sooner than necessary, so we stayed.

The people in the condominium complex were wonderful and very understanding. We attended every event they held and appreciated their helpful and caring attitude. Best of all, they treated my husband like a normal human being, regardless of the strange things he often said and did, and I loved them for it. When I was unable to attend the Ladies' Luncheons because I couldn't leave my husband unattended, they insisted I bring him along as the "token" male. He enjoyed it too, as they spoiled him rotten. He loved the attention and he lapped it up.

One evening, early in our stay there, we attended a tree-trimming party at the condo Club House. I seated Edwin in a comfortable chair by the tree, explaining that I was just going to help the others trim the tree and he could watch. He was very concerned that I might leave him, but I assured him that I was staying right there. Later we had pizza but I noticed that he just folded his up into a big mess. Wanting to help him, I found a sharp knife in the kitchen and proceeded to cut his pizza into bite-size pieces. That was all he needed and he was quite content. Remembering that he'd experienced a similar problem with his meat that same week, it occurred to me that he was no longer able to perform such simple tasks as cutting his food. I think it was also that incident which indicated to others that my husband was not quite normal. At any rate, they accepted the fact with no comment and I appreciated their tact.

It was nice being with other people again, the first time since that fateful night en-route to Florida, and I was glad we'd gone to the party, if only because I had someone else to converse with besides Edwin. He himself didn't enjoy it particularly, but he did admit it "wasn't terrible" either, and it was something different to do. In that respect he appreciated the outing. He would get so bored with himself at home, but he never wanted to do anything either, so I did feel the need to take him out occasionally. It was good for both of us! In fact, even though he'd claim he didn't want to go anywhere, whenever I'd tell him we were going out later, he would ask me over and over when we were leaving. He would even put on his jacket, hours ahead of time, and sit by the door waiting to go.

One evening we went to a Valentine's party at the Club House. Edwin ate very little, but really seemed to enjoy himself nonetheless. After about two hours, however, he became tired and wanted to go home, so we left. Once home he began to rave about how wonderful I was and to tell me how much he loved me. I gave him a big hug and he just hung on to me and cried on my shoulder. He then went on to explain that he was just so moved and impressed by the number of friends we had there, stating that he hadn't had any friends for years before I came along.

The people there in Florida were good too, I had to agree. They really seemed to go out of their way to be nice to Edwin, understanding his condition, but still treating him like a real person. It meant a lot to him, and to me as well. It made things so much easier to take, during those dark and difficult days.

On another one of our outings to a party at the Club House, Edwin was sitting with several of the ladies from the condo and was enjoying their attention. I had gone up to get a plate of food for him, leaving him in their care. Later the ladies related that after I'd left to collect his food, Edwin had commented on his wife saying, "I've got the best!" They thought it was such a sweet thing to say. That was one of the brighter spots of our time there and I know I shall treasure it always.

On the not-so-bright side, it seemed that every night before going to bed we would have a big blow-up and I found it very disturbing. No matter how hard I tried to avoid the situation, it would almost inevitably happen, and I'd end up stressed out and unable to sleep for hours after Edwin would be sleeping peacefully, at least until he'd wake up again for his nocturnal pursuits—but that's another story! It was never anything important, just a total mix-up in communication, and off he'd go on one tangent or another. Every night it was the same. No matter what

I'd say or do, it would be misinterpreted and twisted out of proportion, ending up in a head-on collision! It was virtually impossible to avoid those confrontations—and believe me I tried—as the more I attempted to redirect his ire, the more agitated he would become. When I'd try to keep silent and say nothing, rather than dignify his taunts and questions by answering them which would only have infuriated him further, he would rail at me for being hard-of-hearing! If I tried to calm him down, flatly refusing to fight with him, he would raise his voice even louder and start shouting and yelling! (I often wondered what the poor neighbours must have thought.) Sometimes I'd think I just couldn't take any more myself!

Some time later I gained a whole new perspective on those nightly activities, as we attended a lecture on Alzheimer's disease, sponsored by the Alzheimer's Association of Florida. The main speaker was a doctor from the area, who specialized in the disease, and his presentation was most informative. One of the areas discussed that evening was the subject of Sundowner's Syndrome, a frequent symptom of those suffering from Alzheimer's. As the label suggests, it is a condition that manifests itself as the sun goes down. In this case, it refers to those patients who become increasingly agitated as the day progresses, beginning in the afternoon and culminating in the evening hours, after the sun has set!

That was definitely Edwin's problem! There was no doubt about it! So how could one begin to offset it? Not easily, I assure you, but I did discover a few tricks that helped at least. Apparently the dimming light would trigger their agitation, as they'd become more disorientated the darker it became. Keeping that in mind, every day, before it started to get dark, I would turn on all the lights in the house—and I do mean all! The brighter, the better! I figured if I could convince Edwin that it was still daytime, maybe somehow we could delay the onset of that syndrome, at least for a while. Actually it did help, and I continued the practice of lighting up the house even after we returned home to Canada, and throughout the time we had together.

I might mention here an interesting observation I made during that time. I noticed that Edwin no longer walked upright, as he had always done in the past, but had developed a stooped posture and a shuffling walk. He wouldn't lift his feet any more when he walked, which often caused him to trip or fall. This made it especially difficult for him when walking on grass or uneven surfaces and even on carpet. It was also a problem on vinyl or ceramic floors when he was wearing rubber soles, which would catch, instead of sliding, and precipitate a tumble. The strange thing is though, most of the time he would drag his feet while walking, like an old man, except when he became agitated, as in the evenings at home. Then it was an entirely different story! He'd start pacing the floors, even marching back and forth between the bedroom and the living room, moving quickly and determinedly, something he was incapable of doing, apparently, at any other time. It was almost as if two different people were living in one body!

As the pressure grew, I realized that I needed some sort of break from being with my husband constantly every minute of the day and night, and I started going for long walks very early in the morning, while he was still sleeping. My husband had never been an early riser and it was true even more now, after he wandered around half the night. Suffering with the Sundown Syndrome, as mentioned before, and becoming increasingly agitated in the evenings, he'd eventually wear himself out. Then, completely exhausted, he'd usually fall asleep quite readily. However, he would never stay that way for very long. Two or three hours later he would wake up again, totally confused and disorientated, and would start pacing the floors, dressing and undressing, searching for things and hiding them again, then searching for what he'd just hidden away, convinced that someone had stolen whatever it was. When at last he'd fall asleep once more, usually in the small hours of the morning, I knew he would stay asleep for a few hours at least, having worn himself out with his nocturnal activities. Just to be on the safe side though, I purchased a good set of portable two-way radios, setting one up in the condo and taking the other with me, so I could hear him if he should awaken, and reassure him by talking to him as I hurried home. This worked very well and gave me a much-needed break, along with healthy exercise. Only a few times did he wake up before I arrived back home, and those times the radios proved very effective. He just needed to hear my voice assuring him that I was on my way, and he would be content.

Cleaning Edwin's bathroom one morning, I was appalled at how dirty it had become. He'd never have allowed that to happen before. I also gave him a bath and washed his hair as it was very much overdue and he really needed it. I'd wanted to test him, to see how far he would go if left to his own devices, still not convinced he was unable to do anything for himself, and thinking surely he would know when he needed to wash or change his clothes. I decided to give him one week to try it but the experiment was totally unsuccessful. Fortunately it was a week when we stayed at home, not needing to go out anywhere, for by the end of it I discovered that Edwin had never bathed, even though he'd insisted he had, and had never changed his clothes as well. I couldn't believe it! He was always so clean and fussy about his appearance. How could he have allowed himself to get into such a state? This was definitely not the man I'd known, who took pride in his appearance and was always neat and clean and properly dressed. Obviously, I still hadn't grasped the fact that he really was not responsible for himself, or his actions.

That day I put out clean clothes for him to wear, as I had to do every day thereafter, and then, following his morning coffee, I informed Edwin that he was about to have a bath, over which I was going to preside. Brooking no argument from him, I marched him into the bathroom while I filled the tub. I practically had to lift him into the tub myself, he was so determined not to cooperate, but he finally acquiesced and I managed to get him seated in the warm water. However, once in the tub he just sat there, staring at me resentfully.

"Well, go ahead," I said, "Wash yourself."

"How?" he replied, sitting there in the tub and looking up at me like a lost child.

"Surely you know how!" I said, handing him the washcloth and a bar of soap. "Now go ahead and wash yourself."

He patted himself a few times with the washcloth and then pronounced himself done!

"You might want to try using soap!" I commented dryly, still not able to grasp the situation fully, not wanting to believe what I was witnessing.

Finally, he took the bar of soap and, holding it in his hand, patted his chest with it a few times, just as he had done before with the washcloth. Then, once again he pronounced himself done!

I couldn't believe it! I thought he must have been joking. This couldn't be for real, could it? But it was! Now, as reality set in, I had to face the painful truth: I really had lost my husband and acquired a "man-child" in his place. I could barely contain my tears that day, as they mingled with the wash water, while I proceeded to bathe him myself, still somewhat in shock, but painfully aware of what I'd lost.

Getting him out of the tub after his bath was no small task either, as he could not seem to lift himself, and his feet would slip on the enamel. I later bought a pair of rubber swimming-shoes, which helped considerably, but until then my poor aching back took the brunt of it. Even though he seemed to be so slim, he felt a lot heavier, for lifting him was like lifting a dead weight, since he was unable to help himself at all. (Once home in Canada I invested in a bath chair, which was a great help as well.)

When I managed, finally, to get him out of the tub, I handed him one of the large bath towels to dry himself. However, instead of covering up his soaking wet body, he simply held the huge towel in his hands, delicately drying each hand, slowly and painstakingly, one finger at a time, while he himself stood there, soaking wet, naked, and shivering with the cold. Finally I covered him with the towel, rubbing him dry and putting him out of his misery. I couldn't stand to see him like that, shaking with cold and looking so vulnerable and utterly miserable. What had become of my self-possessed man, so sure of himself and his own abilities? What indeed!

Whenever I would take a bath or shower myself, Edwin would be convinced I was planning to go out somewhere and demand to know where I was going. (After all, why else would I possibly need to bathe?) By the same token, whenever I would clean the condo, he would be convinced that I was expecting company. He hated having company invade his space, or usurp my attention from him, so we never invited anyone over, nor did I ever go anywhere without him. Nevertheless, in both cases he would become paranoid and upset, convinced I wasn't being honest with him.

One of the books I'd read supported two tests that could determine "definite signs" of brain damage, so I decided to try them out. The first test consisted of ten simple questions, where a score of ten indicated a healthy brain. The questions were very basic, such as follows:

Name the Prime Minister of Canada (or the President of the United States).

What day is today?

What year is it?

What is the date today?

What month is it?'

When is your birthday?

None of the questions was any harder than those I've listed but Edwin managed to answer only one correctly. He knew the President of the United States was Clinton, but was unable to name the Prime Minister of Canada. He was also able to remember his birthday, but everything else was beyond him. Of course, later on even his birthday eluded him as the disease progressed. He couldn't even remember what month it was, much less the day or the year. It was really sad. I didn't tell him when his answers were incorrect as he actually thought he'd done well. How could I tell him otherwise?

The other test involved my patting Edwin's cheek, and then his hand, repeatedly, and he was to tell me which of the two I was touching while keeping his eyes closed. More often than not he'd say his hand when I touched his cheek, and vice versa. That was not a good sign! Of course, neither of these tests were absolutely conclusive, so I had no intention of giving up yet, but it did give me a good indication of what I was up against, and I knew it did not augur well for him!

One evening Edwin was upset because we'd run out of his favourite snack. Since the store was right next door to us, I offered to run over and get him some, wanting to encourage him any time he was willing to eat, as he ate so little. However, when I arrived home, not ten minutes later, I found Edwin wandering around outside, totally confused and with no idea where our home was located. He had come out looking for me and was furious that I had gone off without telling him, having completely forgotten, of course, just why I'd gone in the first place. After that he spent the entire evening constantly accusing, demeaning, and belittling me, with caustic comments, cruel accusations, and cutting remarks. My temper and patience were strained to the limit, and I broke down and cried several times, but not even that had any effect on him. I felt so alone! I just did not know what to do any more. I didn't know how much more my patience could endure or how I could withstand any more of his jabs and hurtful thrusts. I was trying so hard but nothing seemed to help, and in my heart I cried out to God. How much longer could I take all this?

Edwin's son phoned one day and Edwin actually agreed to talk with him for a change. He almost sounded normal on the phone, and I wondered what he must have thought after all I'd told him about his dad's condition. Sometimes I didn't know myself what to think! Of course, later on Edwin wouldn't even remember that he'd called, but I'm sure he appreciated it at the time.

At one point, his son asked if we had made lots of friends there in Florida.

Edwin replied, "I don't know. Have we?" he asked, looking at me for confirmation.

"Of course we have," I assured him.

"Yes, we have." He then affirmed on the phone.

During the conversation he also told his son that he liked it here in Florida, one of the reasons being the following, which I'm quoting verbatim.

"You could stop anywhere along the side of the road and buy barrels of booze, and no one thought anything of it!"

(I sure hope he didn't think we were actually buying "barrels of booze"!) It was strange sometimes how Edwin would express himself, and I often wondered what was running through his head, in reality, at times like that. Guess I'll never know!

One day during one of his more lucid moments, Edwin confessed to me that every time he'd doze off, he would wake up totally disorientated, but that the minute he'd see me he would know that everything was all right. As much as I could appreciate his complete dependence on me to make his world all right, it could be quite a burden. I couldn't even step out to the store, or the mailbox, or the garbage disposal bin, without him panicking. I would carefully explain where I was going, and I'd never be gone more than a few minutes at most, but even in that short time he would forget where I was or even that I'd gone. Then he would panic and become furious at me when I returned, convinced I'd been gone for hours.

I tried solving this issue by writing a short note for him, telling him where I was when I had to step out for the mail etc. I thought this was a great idea but unfortunately it backfired on me. When I tried telling him where I was going, and giving him a note to confirm where I'd be, he would then panic before I left, as the note made him think my going out was a big deal and I was never coming back. I couldn't win, no matter what I did, but I just kept on trying.

During those first few months I was becoming increasingly concerned over Edwin's physical health, not to mention his mental stability. He seemed to be failing rapidly, physically as well as mentally. Finding it difficult even to get himself out of a chair, he would sometimes make two or three attempts before accomplishing it. He would also lose his balance a lot, for no apparent reason; not only when he was walking, but even when he'd just be standing in one place, and I was constantly on edge. At times he seemed to resent my attempts to help, so I'd try to let him do things for himself whenever possible, but often I'd end up having to do them for him in the end.

At least I knew it wasn't being in Florida that was causing his problems. He loved it there, in spite of all his complaining. In fact, he expressed that sentiment countless times while we were there—and even after we'd gone home. One day he said to me that every morning in Florida he would wake up thinking it was too good to be true. At one point, early in our sojourn, he asked me how many days we had left there and I told him not to worry as we were still counting in months. He seemed amazed to realize it was still only December.

I said, "Of course it is! December can't be over until we've had Christmas and we haven't had Christmas yet!"

He was genuinely surprised, thinking that Christmas was already just a memory, finished with a long time ago. (You'd think he would have wondered why we still had our Christmas tree in the living room.)

Another thing I noticed as time progressed was Edwin's increasing difficulty in using his left arm or hand, either in dressing or eating. He would feed himself with his right hand, but could not manage a fork and knife together. This was especially noteworthy as he had always eaten his meals with a knife and fork in the past—even pizza or a hamburger. He would make an exception when it came to eating a sandwich, but even then he would use cutlery if possible. Fingers were never an option with him, so when it became impossible for him to pick up something with just his fork, he would get frustrated and give up in disgust, not eating it at all, rather than use his fingers. Also, buttons and shoelaces, requiring two hands, became almost impossible for him over time. I managed to find him some shoes with Velcro closures instead of laces, and he was very pleased with them. The rest of his shoes I converted to elastic laces, which also helped.

When it came to mealtimes, I would find it frustrating watching Edwin eat. He was so slow and methodical; his movements so studied, yet uncertain. He had increasing difficulty managing his utensils as I mentioned before, but using his fingers was abhorrent to him. (Must have been his proper British background!) In the course of a meal, if he spilled food on himself (heaven forbid!), he would get mad at me, saying I distracted him when I talked at the table, so for the most part we were forced to eat in silence.

I was very thankful for the books I had been studying, as they helped me, in no small way, to grasp the underlying reasons for much of his behaviour. It also helped to keep me from getting unduly upset at what used to appear as slurs to myself, as I seemed to be the recipient of so much blame from my husband. In actuality, he was simply frustrated with himself and his inability to function as normal.

Also in regard to eating, if I served anything which involved a dip, such as veggies and dip or any other finger-foods, he would have to ask me, before each bite, just what he was supposed to do with it and how he was supposed to eat it. As it was, I would cut up all his food for him. He'd eat more if he didn't have to struggle with it, and it would be too late to help him after he'd struggled with anything, as by then he'd have lost his appetite due to frustration, and would refuse to eat any more at all.

His favourite meal was lunch. At least that's when he would eat the most, not that he ever ate a lot any more. It usually consisted of sandwiches made with cold cuts, pickles, and mustard or mayonnaise. He always enjoyed making his own sandwich so I'd put all the ingredients on the table and let him do his own thing. The day arrived, however, when even that became too much for him. Instead of making a normal sandwich, he put two slices of bread together, with the cold cuts and mayonnaise on top. What a mess! He had a very difficult time eating it, since he always hated messing his fingers, but he never realized that he had done anything wrong. From that point on he'd find even more bizarre ways to make his sandwiches until I had to take over and make them myself.

As the disease progressed, he ate less and less and it was a challenge trying to find foods that he enjoyed and would eat at all. One of his favourite restaurants was the Red Lobster so I would take him there fairly often, as he'd eat more on those occasions than at any other time. On one such visit he fussed because there were no shrimps on his salad. I explained that he never had shrimp on his salad but that the shrimp would be on his dinner plate. He was all right after that but it seemed that even such simple things would all get muddled in his mind.

When we arrived home, the neighbour's dog was barking. I guess we must have disturbed it, as another dog started barking as well. At any rate, after that I had to sit through a long dissertation about "dogs sitting at the dinner table, eating shrimp and disturbing everyone by barking and barking!" He simply mixed all his experiences together until they became one big story in his imagination, and he'd be convinced they were true.

Another idiosyncrasy involving restaurants occurred whenever we were given linen napkins, as Edwin would always want to take his home with him. He'd usually stuff it into his pocket, but as they were bulky, it was easy to spot. It became a little trickier later on when he discovered the "neat pocket" in the front of his trousers. He thought that was a great little hidey-hole and would stuff all sorts of things down there, including his handkerchief! It could be quite embarrassing, especially when he opened up his fly in public, either to stuff something in it or to search for something he thought should be there! There were even times when he'd half undress himself in public, removing articles of clothing, while looking for his handkerchief or anything else he couldn't find. I didn't dare let him out of my sight for long, as I could never be sure what he might do. (I must say there was never anything boring about this disease!)

At any rate, he could be quite unpredictable at times and I never knew what to expect next. One thing that helped to keep me going, though, was a sense of humour. There were times when I really didn't know whether to laugh or cry—and I did both, believe me. I'd often think of the line from a song that says, "It's my party, and I'll cry if I want to," but I really didn't want to cry all the time. It didn't help anyway, just left me feeling drained and exhausted, so I tried desperately, to hang on to my sense of humour. That was difficult at the best of times, but so often it was simply a case of "if I didn't laugh, I'd cry." Some of the things he did and said were funny—even if they were also sad—and I tried to see the humorous side as much as possible, if only to keep my sanity.

I can remember hearing an excerpt from a poem called "Solitude" in my childhood. It was written by Ella Wheeler Wilcox and seemed appropriate for my situation:

Laugh, and the world laughs with you;
Weep, and you weep alone;
For the sad old earth must borrow its mirth,
But has trouble enough of its own.

I knew what it was to cry alone! I would never wish that on anyone else. No one needs to feel so alone, as I did. There is help out there, but you have to go after it yourself. No one can do it for you—no one, but you! One of the hardest things to do in life is to admit defeat, to admit that you can't do something by yourself, that you need help. Until we recognize the fact that we can't do something alone, that we do need help, there is no reprieve. Swallow your pride, or whatever it is that is holding you back, and start searching for all the help lines available to you. The government has some marvellous agencies offering various types of help and service, and those, along with the Alzheimer's Society and related organizations and support groups, can make all the difference in the world to someone struggling with Alzheimer's disease in a loved one. Don't wait until it's too late! Don't wait until your health breaks down, your spirit is broken, or your nerves shot. If you want to help your loved one, you must first learn to help yourself. I had to learn this for myself—the hard way—and I would implore you to accept it from one who knows, someone who's been there! There is help for you out there! Go and find it, avail yourself of it, and help your loved one—even as you help yourself!

The Third Man Theme

One day Edwin began talking about the "other brother," asking what had happened to him. I had no idea to whom he was referring and asked him to explain. He then insisted there was another man living with us in the condo, the same man who had driven down to Florida with us in the car. I still didn't understand and he became most upset with me.

"You know!" he said, rather crossly. "There are usually three of us together, two men and one woman. You're the woman but who is the other man?"

I was at a loss to answer him but he was convinced the other man existed and that I should know what his name was.

On our way down to Florida, Edwin had often referred to the "other man" travelling with us. I'd just laughed and stated the obvious, that there was no room in the car for anyone else as we were loaded to the hilt with luggage. However, he continued to insist that another man had been sitting in the back seat all the way there. I had actually forgotten all about that, until this conversation first came up in Florida, but I still had no idea who or what he was talking about. (Too bad there wasn't someone else around. I could really have used some help with Edwin once in awhile!) On a similar subject, he used to ask me constantly who lived out on our patio, as though that door led to another unit entirely, yet we spent a good part of our day out there, enjoying the warmth and the sunshine.

A few months later I actually discovered just who the "other man" was, the one who supposedly travelled with us to Florida and back, and usually lived in our home with us. One of the doctors explained him as being "the man in the mirror." Just as Edwin did not always recognize me or people he used to know, so too he didn't even recognize himself! Thus his own reflection in the mirror, looking back at him, had to be another man, one he felt he should know but couldn't quite place. Apparently this phenomenon is quite common in Alzheimer's disease. It made sense too, as the car was so loaded with luggage, driving down to Florida, that I was unable to use the rear view mirror as such, and had to depend on the side mirrors. Therefore, I set the rear view mirror to cover the usual blind spot on the passenger side of the car. It actually worked quite well for me, but I guess that also enabled Edwin to see his own image looking back at him, if he wasn't looking out of the window. That would explain his supposedly seeing someone sitting in the back of the car. It was his own reflection, which he did not recognize. At least it was nice to have one mystery solved!

One afternoon while we were sitting out on the patio enjoying the lovely Florida weather, Edwin told me out of the blue, that I was "idyllic." It was a nice compliment, one I still savour, but I marveled at his choice of words. With Alzheimer's disease, patients lose their ability to express themselves in words, as their vocabulary shrinks considerably. However, for Edwin it was not as great a problem as for others in his situation, since being educated in Britain, and from the "old school," as it were, he had always enjoyed an amazing vocabulary. Normally he would take three sentences to say what the rest of us would say in one, but his speech was charming and poetic. In fact, it was one of the things I'd always loved about him, his ability to express himself so eloquently. Thus, even with the dementia slowly but inexorably robbing him of his abilities, he still had a large store of words to draw from, giving him an advantage that most sufferers of the disease did not enjoy, and enabling him to express himself much longer than most during the course of the disease.

Along with his verbal skills, there was another area that caught my attention, insofar as Edwin's abilities were concerned. This involved his social skills, which actually seemed to be improving rather than regressing, at least at that early stage. Before Alzheimer's disease struck him down, Edwin really didn't care what people thought of him, so at times he didn't even try to be sociable if he didn't feel like it. During those months in Florida it was just the opposite, as it seemed he was really trying to be sociable, at times anyway. He would often amaze me with his attempts to please, smiling and making comments and acting almost normal, if I didn't know better. Almost, of course, is the operative word. Unfortunately this did not apply at home where it obviously did not matter how he behaved, or perhaps he just felt he could relax there, but away from home he became another person entirely.

One evening, friends of ours invited us to join them at a restaurant for dinner. I said I'd call them back and mentioned the invitation to Edwin. He said no, he didn't want to go and was adamant in his refusal. He liked eating out, but only with me alone. Trying to convince him otherwise, I mentioned the fact that he was always so good when he was out with other people so I thought he enjoyed it. He then went on to explain that he was tired of lying, and that when he was with other people it was all a big lie, because he couldn't say what he really wanted to say. I was surprised at this and asked him why he couldn't say what he wanted to say.

He replied, "I've learned in the business that you always have to lie. That's the only way you can get along with people!"

Needless to say, we didn't go! However, his comment was a real revelation to me. I certainly didn't want to make things any more difficult for him than they were, so I resolved, then and there, not to make any more plans for the future, whenever feasible. I kept to this plan as much as possible too, but there were occasions when we had no choice, though I tried to consider his feelings and make things as easy on him as I possibly could. Interestingly enough, though, I noticed that whenever we did plan to go out somewhere, he actually appeared eager to go, which did seem to belie his claim to the contrary.

For instance, one day I had an appointment to get my hair cut, which was long overdue, I might add. I was able to cut Edwin's hair myself but I still had to go out to get mine done. I explained where we were going and told him that we didn't have to leave the house until 11 a.m. However, he was dressed and ready to go by 10 a.m. and sat there waiting for me, with his jacket and hat on, for one whole hour. He stayed right by the front door too, the entire time. Perhaps he was afraid I'd leave without him. Before we left I did have to remove his jacket to change his vest, which was inside out, and I also had to zip his fly, but that was a minor detail. The important thing was that he was ready and eager to go with me, and even at the salon he was content to sit for over an hour, waiting for me while I had my hair done. For someone who swore he didn't want to go anywhere, he sure was eager to go whenever we did go out. In fact, I finally had to stop letting him know in advance when we were going anywhere, opting instead to telling him at the last minute, for otherwise he would be dressed and waiting in the morning, ready to go on an outing planned for that evening. I was glad he was so pleased to be going, but sometimes he'd drive me crazy, asking over and over, every ten minutes throughout the day, when we were leaving. What I wouldn't have given for a happy medium, but it was always all or nothing with him!

When bedtime came each night, he would ask again where he should sleep, insisting that I kept on changing the location. I'd also have to show him where his bathroom was located and without fail he'd claim that he'd never been there before, even though he'd used that same bathroom every day since we'd been there. When I'd point this out to him he'd deny it vigorously, claiming that I was making it up. In fact, all day long it would be the same. I was the problem, not him! I was inventing all these stories to confuse him but he couldn't be fooled—oh no, not him! He would just talk a lot of nonsense, making up wonderful stories and filling them in with facts, names, and places, things that actually existed, but just not in the jumbled mix he'd conceived in his own mind. Throughout all his stories though, one thread was paramount, his rampant paranoia that everything and everybody was out to get him!

Some days he would be much more docile than others and not so cuttingly cruel. I would cherish those days, knowing they would not last, but trying to use them to mend my own bruised ego. It was so hard not to take his comments personally, and at times I'd feel very hurt and confused myself, wondering why he would become so mean and cruel when all I did was try to help him.

Later I learned that it was fear that drove him. Even normal people will lash out in anger when driven by fear. How could we expect less in someone no longer in control of his emotions? Realizing that things were not right with him, yet unwilling to admit it, and unable to control the situation, he would lash out at anyone near him. Alzheimer's patients can become very hostile at times, especially to the care-giver, who is often seen as the enemy, and Edwin was no exception. Not being able to accept the blame themselves, they lash out at others, usually those closest to them. Actually, that is one area of the disease which sets apart those with Alzheimer's from people merely suffering memory loss associated with advancing age. Whereas a person merely suffering from age related lapses of memory will readily acknowledge the problem and even request help in recalling information, the Alzheimer's patient will attempt to compensate for the lapse by denying its existence and blaming someone else.

Sometimes I would take Edwin to a place he'd been before, and he would recognize the fact that he had been there in the past, as it would seem vaguely familiar to him. However, even if he'd been there only the day before, he would insist that it had been a long time ago, even years perhaps, if he remembered it at all. Obviously some of his recollections were still there, though very dim, and becoming dimmer with each passing day.

As time progressed, Edwin could no longer get any satisfaction out of reading the daily newspaper, once a longstanding habit with him. He would often pretend to do so, or perhaps he thought he really was reading it, but the paper could just as easily be upside down and he wouldn't realize it. Reading books also became impossible for him, as well as watching TV. He was just too restless and agitated most of the time, pacing back and forth, unable to sit down for any length of time, except when he would doze off, which was becoming less and less frequent. Some evenings however, he would enjoy cuddling up on the couch, watching the pictures on the television with me, though not actually following any sequence or program. Then he'd pick out the odd words, or a picture, and home in on that subject, usually to my dismay. For example, if the news commentator mentioned a snowstorm in another state, or up in Canada, Edwin would then warn me to stay inside because he was convinced there was a storm outside and the snow was deep and cold. This was in Florida when the temperature was in the 80's!

Another time he would hear about a war somewhere in the world, or an act of war, and would immediately become terrified that the 'Bully Boys' were going to break down our door. (Apparently the Bully Boys were gangs of rough necks back in Britain, who preyed on others and robbed them.)

One evening, while watching TV, he asked me the following question:

"How long do we have to keep making payments?" I asked him what payments he was talking about and he replied somewhat irritably.

"To the man on the TV of course."

Sometimes he would make me feel stupid for not knowing what he was talking about, like I should know, but I had no way of knowing, if I couldn't make the connection. It finally came to the point that I decided it was best to curtail his TV watching. He just couldn't handle it any more. He couldn't follow the sequence of events on the programs—not even his favourite ones—and would become extremely agitated. When he did understand something that was said he'd usually take it literally, as it related to him, and more trouble would erupt. Even the news and weather would evoke severe reactions, as he'd be convinced that snowstorms, hurricanes, tornadoes, earthquakes, and whatever else they talked about, were happening to him right then and there, and there was no convincing him otherwise. If it was on the TV then it must be real!

Speaking of watching TV, I would also find that most of the times Edwin felt inclined to talk to me at any length were when I was trying to listen to something on the television. The rest of the time he would just sit there staring into space and barely responding, if at all, when I would speak to him. However, as soon as I'd turn on the TV he'd decide to talk! I'm not sure if he was just being ornery, or jealous for my attention, or if the TV actually stimulated him to talk. Whatever it was, it could be very frustrating, so I tried to avoid setting my own agenda. I figured that if I didn't set my heart on watching a certain program, then I couldn't be disappointed or upset if I missed it. That was my theory anyway and it did help; when I followed my own advice, that is!

One evening there was a comedy on TV that I had wanted to see for some time. I didn't usually insist on having my own way but there was nothing else worth watching anyway, and I really wanted to see that movie, so I decided to watch it. I tried to get Edwin to sit with me and cuddle up on the couch the way he enjoyed, but that night he was in one of his ugly moods and refused to join me at all. I tried to be patient with him but he could be so exasperating at those times.

He asked me, "Just what am I supposed to do while you're watching that garbage?"

I replied, somewhat tersely, "Well you don't usually do anything anyway so what's the difference?" As you can see, I was somewhat upset myself by that time. Anyway, he got mad and stomped off to bed. For a while I was relieved that he'd gone but then my conscience got the better of me and I went to tuck him in. Finding the bedroom door closed, I opened it and went in to kiss him good night and see if he needed anything. On leaving, I closed the door again behind me. A few minutes later he marched out into the living room, angry with me for closing the door, and demanding to know what was on TV that I didn't want him to watch? What was I trying to hide from him anyway? It would amaze me constantly, how he could turn things around and twist them totally out of context. We could enjoy such nice times together and then he would ruin it all with his bitter, vitriolic tirades and sarcasm. I seemed to live with a knot in my stomach most of the time those days, afraid to do or say anything that would trigger an eruption from him. He was like a simmering volcano just beneath the surface, and I was slowly becoming a nervous wreck!

One morning we had a merry little hunt for Edwin's teeth, finally locating them in the bedroom dresser drawer. (Other times he would find even more ingenious places to hide them.) That day we also had to search for his razor, which ultimately we discovered hiding beneath his underwear. (Of course! Why didn't I think of that?) Then followed a search for his hearing aid. That was a tougher challenge, but it turned up at last, well wrapped in Kleenex, resting in an ashtray in one of his drawers. Of course the Kleenex put us off the trail at first, but in time that was to become his signature activity, wrapping things up in Kleenex before hiding them away. Unfortunately a number of his possessions ended up in the garbage that way as well.

At that point in time I devised a way to make things a little easier, for both of us! (I figured I was finally getting smart in my old age, or desperate! Whatever!) At any rate, to preserve my sanity (and my feet), I printed notes to tape up all over the house, explaining where everything was and where they should go. I printed the notes in large capital letters, keeping them as simple as possible so that he would have no trouble understanding them. For example, a note on his bedside table read YOUR HEARING AID GOES IN THIS DISH AT NIGHT. I included descriptions of where to put, and where to find, his razor, teeth, pyjamas, socks, shorts, undershirts, etc., and kept each item in separate drawers to simplify his search. I also printed out instructions on how to find his bedroom, the bathroom, the front door, the patio door and so on. Interestingly enough, I never had to show him where the kitchen was located. He just knew, instinctively! (I wonder what that tells us, if anything?) I also labelled each door, indicating which room it was. This seemed rather bizarre, even as I did it, but it actually helped a lot and I think even Edwin appreciated the sense of independence it generated for him. Of course I had to encourage him to read the notes many times, when he would start asking where things were or where he should go, but he enjoyed being able to find things for himself, and the notes helped immensely. There was still some confusion of course, but it improved things overall, and each time Edwin would read a note it was—for him anyway—as though he were reading it for the first time, each day!

When certain items disappeared I would often find them in Edwin's pockets. Of course, without fail, he'd insist that he hadn't put them there. The same applied when we'd find things of his that were missing, usually hidden away in some unique hiding place. Of course he never did that either! (That was some "gremlin" we had in our house!)

One evening when we went out for supper, Edwin needed a toothpick after the meal, so I loaned him mine. It was a very special, reusable, plastic one and I only had three of them. I'd given my husband one to keep in his pocket, which he'd obviously misplaced, and I didn't want to lose mine too, so on arriving back home I asked him to return the one I'd loaned him. He couldn't find it as it wasn't in his shirt pocket, but when I searched his jacket I found it there, along with the one I'd given him previously. Of course he insisted he hadn't put either of them in that location but I was just glad to get them back and once again replaced his in his shirt pocket, showing him that I was putting it there, where he was supposed to keep it.

A few minutes later he came to me and said, "I told you I put it in my shirt pocket!" So saying, he pulled the toothpick out of his pocket, exclaiming, "See! Here it is!"

"Of course it's there," I said. "I just put it in there as I told you!"

He then insisted that it had been there all along, even though he'd searched the pocket himself earlier, looking for it. There was no point in arguing, of course, but it sure could be frustrating, especially when he would not give up until I'd conceded that he was right. I learned a lot of lessons in humility those days!

For dinner one night I cooked a lovely Chicken Kiev with mixed vegetables and salad. Edwin really loved it, eating more than usual, which pleased me, and we enjoyed a pleasant, leisurely meal with candles on the table, quiet music, and lots of atmosphere. What more could you want? However, an hour later Edwin asked me what I'd had for dinner! I told him that I'd had the same food that he did but he wanted to know what we'd eaten, so I recounted a description of our lovely meal to him.

Then he asked, "What did the children have for dinner?"

I said, "What children?"

He got very upset at that and said, "Don't tell me there were no children, because I saw them. They were right here in our living room, all dressed up!"

Another day poor Edwin tried for over an hour to put a new film in his camera. I offered to help but he flatly refused. Later he finally admitted to needing help but by then he'd run the film right through, so there was no end left to thread. (Loading a film was like breathing to a photographer like him, his stock-in-trade until then, and there he was, no longer able to accomplish even this simple task.) Thinking to help him, I opened a new box of film to put into his camera, but he insisted that the film was already in the camera. I then opened the camera to show him it was empty, but then he asked me why I had removed the film from the camera. I told him I hadn't removed it but he insisted that I had, pointing to the new film in my hand.

"Yes you did!" he said. "There it is, there in your hand!"

Such interplay was typical those days, and would go on and on if I didn't stop it. To do so I'd just have to swallow my pride and admit to whatever he'd accused me of doing. Then I'd have to listen to him ranting and raving about how he was right and I was wrong and he knew best, ad nauseam! However, it was still better than arguing!

Later on he ruined another film, while trying to remove it from his camera. He still could not accept the fact that he was the problem though, and blamed it on the camera. I had let him take lots of photographs to that point, even encouraged him to do so, as it gave him an interest and it was a hobby he'd always enjoyed. However, by then I was beginning to think it was about time for him to stop, especially since he would also become very frustrated when none of his pictures turned out right. That day he was determined to go to the photo shop in order to talk to the man about his camera. He wouldn't give up and, finally, I just had to sit back and let him do his thing. However, as it turned out, he couldn't find the front door of our house and I certainly wasn't going to show him where it was. Thus, after searching for a time, becoming more and more frustrated and indignant all the while, he eventually forgot what he was intending to do in the first place and gave up. I would feel so sorry for him— and helpless as well—yet at times like that it was almost funny! Almost...but who felt like laughing?

The last few days of our stay in Florida I was kept busy cleaning the condo: vacuuming the floors, washing the walls and woodwork and preparing to leave the place in perfect condition for the next renters. Edwin followed me about the entire time, constantly underfoot, just like a puppy dog. In fact, often I would have to move him— physically—out of the way so I could vacuum around him but he continued to stay close by me the entire time. He never lifted a finger to help of course, but he never let me out of his sight! It was very difficult to work under those circumstances, and frustrating too, but there was nothing I could do about it, so I carried on.

Three days before leaving he had another bad tumble. He was trying to get into his chair at the dinner table and fell over backwards with the chair, hitting his head on the corner of the wall. It really scared me as I was in the kitchen and couldn't get to him in time, but fortunately he was okay. He seemed to have a hard head if nothing else! It always scared me when he'd fall, and that one was especially frightening, but I had to admire his resilience. Two days later he had another fall, that time into the bushes, trying to navigate the front walk. I was loading the car for our trip home and had my arms full. When I looked back he was lying in the bushes. He sustained a few scratches but nothing serious. (I'm not sure about the bushes!)

Thus we maintained the status quo and managed to keep our heads above water, as it were, while remaining in Florida for the rest of the winter; but the day finally dawned when we had to leave and return to Canada. It was a challenge and I was dreading it. This time I was determined, however, to make the journey as easy as possible on my husband, deciding to take four days and three nights to drive it, instead of rushing. For the most part it was uneventful, except for two occasions when he opened the car door while I was driving. Unfortunately our car did not have child-safe locks so it was not possible to keep him from unlocking his door by turning the handle. Also the seat belts were attached to the door so it was doubly frightening as I would hang on to him with one hand and try to steer the car to the side of the road with the other. Needless to say, I soon traded in that car for one with better safety devices and seat belts, since he did the same thing again after arriving home. Meanwhile, I was just concentrating on getting home—in one piece!

During the journey home Edwin asked me, "Now tell me, just what exactly are we going to be doing, once we get wherever we're supposed to be going?"

I explained that we were going home, and his response was surprising.

"What exactly do you mean by home?" he asked.

He really had no concept any more of where we were, where we'd been, or where we were going.

At lunch in the restaurant, he picked up a forkful of scrambled eggs and asked, "Is this fried tomatoes?" (I don't even think he saw the movie!)

Trying to make the journey as easy as possible for Edwin, I stopped early each night at the motel and would take him for a nice walk before dinner, to exercise his legs after sitting all day. Unfortunately, my plans to make the evenings relaxing for him did not materialize, as each night he would be crabby and irritable and nothing would please him, no matter what I did.

One evening, when he took out his hearing aid to go to bed, he decided to fill the dish with water.

"I wanted to keep my hearing aid from drying out." he explained later, when I asked him why he'd done it.

Fortunately, I caught it right away and raced to dump out the water, removing the battery to dry, before it was ruined. Honestly, I just never knew what he was going to do next! He would also keep trying to hide everything, finding unique places to store them, so each morning before leaving the motel I'd have to check out all the hiding places very carefully, ensuring that nothing was left behind or forgotten.

Once we had crossed over the border into Canada, the first thing I did was to stop for gas. Most border towns are old and run down and that place was no exception.

Edwin looked around him and commented, "If this is where we live, we'll have to do something about getting out of here right away!"

When we arrived at our house, after taking four full days en route, Edwin was convinced that we had just left Florida that same morning and even related the same to his son, when we called to let him know we were home. Fortunately, however, he liked his "new" home! Even if he didn't remember it consciously, I'm sure it must have felt familiar to him, or comfortable, on some unconscious level. I just can't imagine him forgetting it entirely, not after thirty-nine years in the same place.

It was so good to be back home, back in our own country, and back in our own house. However, in my ignorance I'd convinced myself that things would get better once we were home again. But I was wrong, very, very wrong, as I was to learn to my disappointment and dismay all too soon after our return.

Incidentally, in case you were wondering, yes the "third man" did return to Canada with us. In fact, he became firmly ensconced as a permanent member of our household. It was either that, or get rid of all the mirrors in the house, but I didn't mind, not after finding out his identity. Since I had to take care of one man, what was one more?

In Retrospect

Once back in Canada I set up appointments with Edwin's doctor and specialists to have him properly tested and diagnosed, but it was no surprise when he was finally pronounced to be suffering from Alzheimer's disease. The only thing that still confused me about his case was the apparent sudden onset of the disease, and I asked the doctor about it. He explained that it only appeared to be sudden, a frequent occurrence among "snow birds," since the patient is uprooted from their familiar surroundings and it becomes harder for them to "pretend," or put on an act. In Alzheimer's disease the last thing to go is the social skills, so even though they are aware that something is terribly wrong, they are able to hide it—sometimes for a long time—simply by using conditioned or memorized responses, ingrained from childhood. Since people tend not to delve deeper into others' motives or reasons, by using these methods a person can hide their condition indefinitely, or at least until their actions become truly bizarre.

This was certainly true with my husband, as he actually became more sociable with the Alzheimer's disease than he ever was before. He didn't care what people thought of him before, for the most part, but changed quite radically in that department during his illness. A favourite response of his became the expression, "I'm very happy for you," and he used it extensively. People really thought he meant it and was responding to their comments. It actually worked very well for him too, until the day a lady told him of her mother having just died. Only then did it become apparent that he was using a conditioned response and not really understanding what was said to him at all.

Actually, it was rather embarrassing to hear him say to the grieving person, "I'm very happy for you!"

"It's like water dripping into a bucket": so the doctor explained it to me. "It's not really that noticeable while it's just dripping, but once the bucket is full, it overflows, becoming very obvious to everyone. Thereafter it continues to overflow and the damage is done."

In retrospect, I had to admit that there had been many indications of his advancing condition, but none of them in themselves were conclusive. It was only as you put them all together that you actually saw the signs. At any rate, hindsight is always much clearer than foresight, and in a sense I guess we were all in denial as well. No one wants to believe something negative that is happening, either to them or to the ones they love, myself most of all. Now, of course, I can *only* look back as there *is* no future, at least not for us.

I should explain further at this juncture, that one phenomenon I noticed throughout the nightmare in Florida, was the dramatic change for the better in Edwin's behaviour during the times when we were out in public. It was like a transformation, and it would amaze me each time it happened. At first I would rejoice in it, thinking he was improving, until I realized it only lasted while we were out, and would end abruptly the minute we returned home. It was almost as though he was putting on an act, and in a sense I guess he was, as he became an entirely different person. He would actually be transformed from the obsessive, abusive man he had recently become, into a sweet, compliant, and taciturn person in public, albeit totally reliant on me, almost to the point of abject dependency. He would still have moments of relapse, but they would not last for long, at least at that early stage of the disease. Later on the differences in him were not as definitive or stark, but he still seemed to make the effort, at least in public.

I learned some time later, that such behaviour is actually quite normal in Alzheimer's disease. As I mentioned before, the last thing to go is the social skills, the ability to act in public according to the social graces learned, usually, as a young child. In fact, it is in this way that so many patients actually manage to hide the fact of their disease for as long as they do. Most people, socially, do not look for the meaning behind the words spoken, as they too engage in verbal platitudes and so do not recognize—or wish to recognize—their insincerity reflected in others. "How are you today?" and "I'm fine, thank you," become just words and nothing more: socially accepted platitudes, observing the niceties of society. Who wants to hear the truth?

"Well, I'm really not fine at all! My back hurts, my brain is all messed up, I can't remember anything anymore, and just who are you anyway? I don't remember your name or even if I know you at all."

I don't think so!

Looking back, I can see so many signs signalling the onset of this disease, but at the time I just made excuses for him. After all, forgetfulness does accompany advancing age, and I certainly had my times of forgetfulness as well. If I saw any signs in him, I saw them just as much in myself, and no one wants to admit to such things, least of all myself. I used to take pride in my good memory, but now it's not nearly as sharp as it used to be, though one does learn to compensate. You start making lists, writing things down, consciously committing things to memory. Why should my husband be any different? Perhaps if I refused to see the signs in him, I wouldn't have to face them in myself. Who knows? At any rate I closed my eyes to the possibility of anything being amiss. When it started to take him the whole day to write the cheques to pay his monthly bills, I should have suspected something, but then again, not necessarily. Not everyone is good with math. I offered to help and was encouraged by him to take over the accounting, since it was easier for me. It made me feel needed and useful so I did it, gladly.

Next he started becoming paranoid, constantly worrying that someone was out to get him or trying to steal his money or his precious camera, and on and on. I was no longer allowed to open the curtains, as someone might be looking in, so I had to learn to live in a dark house—but it was lovely and cool in the summertime. Then too, if anyone came to the door, he would always accompany me to answer it in order to protect me from harm—but it was nice to feel protected and to know that he cared enough to do so. Thus I continued to make excuses for his behaviour.

One incident that might have presaged his advancing condition was his failure, on more than one occasion, to place the shower curtain inside the tub before taking a shower. Unfortunately this recurring error caused the water to leak into the basement, precipitating my need to re-caulk the floor tiles in the bathroom. However, I tended to excuse this as being quite understandably a "male" thing, since men invariably had other more important things on their minds, and I actually blamed myself for having placed the curtain on the outside of the tub in the first place, putting aesthetics before practicality. After that I adjusted the curtain, rather than blaming him for carelessness, feeling that I probably could have made the same mistake quite easily myself if I wasn't paying attention.

Another thing I noticed was his tendency to compulsive behaviour, at least in regard to certain things. For instance, his camera was a major focus for him. Having been a professional photographer, his camera was his most important possession. He loved photography, as do I, and we would take every opportunity to go on photographic excursions whenever and wherever possible, as weather and circumstances would allow. This included driving up north for the fall colours, going on a major trip, or just going to the park. In any event, the camera was always packed and ready to go at a moment's notice. However, when it was not feasible to take photos, he was still obsessed with his camera, making sure it was clean and ready to go at all times. This in itself would not have been alarming, but for the fact that he would actually dismantle his camera completely, once or twice in any given day, ensuring that all the parts were still there. Then he would carefully reassemble it again; painstakingly wrapping all the extra lenses and pieces, and packing them back into his camera bag, only to repeat the entire process all over again the very next day.

This repetitive behaviour used to drive me crazy, and I even tried putting his camera away in the closet at times, hoping he'd forget about it, but he never did. Eventually I just accepted it as his fetish, realizing that at least it gave him something to do. I knew this behaviour was not exactly normal, but in his case I put it down to boredom and tried to encourage him to find other pursuits and avenues of interest, but never with much success.

Gardening was something I really enjoyed doing and Edwin would often come out to join me as I worked. Realizing the fresh air and the exercise were also good for him, I encouraged his participation in working around the yard. He seemed to enjoy it and was always very eager to help. One day, having noticed me spraying the weeds on the driveway with "Roundup" (a weed-killer which kills everything in its path), Edwin decided to do the same for our lawn. Without my knowing it, he took the container and very carefully sprayed each and every weed in our yard, front and back. A couple of days later I was shocked to discover that our entire lawn was dotted with large, white circles of dead grass. I couldn't imagine what had caused such a phenomenon, having never seen anything like it before. It was bizarre! However, then I discovered the empty bottle of Roundup and it dawned on me what had happened. Poor Edwin readily confessed, convinced at the time that he was being helpful, and I didn't have the heart to get mad at him. In fact, I thanked him for trying to help. However, I also entreated him never to do it again. At any rate, all that summer we had a polka-dot lawn. It was really rather unique! Was that a manifestation of his encroaching disease? Quite possibly it was, but then again, who doesn't make mistakes? He didn't know that product was only for using on paths and driveways. I suppose he could have read the instructions—but he didn't. At any rate I just thought it was an honest mistake at the time.

Another minor incident involved our purchasing a new VCR, since the old one had given up the ghost, and Edwin insisted he wanted one where you could program it with numbers, rather than having to insert the time and day whenever you wanted to record something. However, after having the new machine for two weeks, Edwin was still unable to use it, completely confused and perplexed by the intricacies of the new video player. I tried making a list of simple instructions for him, but nothing helped. It was totally beyond his expertise, something I found quite surprising, given his background in electronics. However, I realized that a lot of things had changed in regard to modern technology in recent years, so again I made excuses for him. As it was, I decided the new VCR wasn't worth the money, since Edwin couldn't use it anyway, so I returned it to the store and had the old one fixed. It ended up lasting for several more years too, amazingly enough, as it was pretty old already.

Another change in him involved our relationship, and this change did concern me as he became very possessive and almost jealous of any time I spent away from him. Once every two weeks I used to go out for an afternoon by myself, when I'd conduct some business, have lunch with my friends, have my nails or hair done, or sometimes even go to a movie with my girlfriend. Poor Edwin, who used to encourage me in the past to go and spend time with my friends, actually began to resent any time I was away from him, and I'd have to call him several times during the afternoon to assure him I was fine. If I didn't call he'd start worrying about me, but on the other hand it was nice having someone to care. When I'd return from my bi-weekly afternoon away, however, he would be in a really sulky mood, thus making my home-coming something to endure, rather than something to anticipate. After awhile he started his sulking the day before I'd go out, continuing to sulk the day after as well. It got to the point where I questioned whether it was worth the effort of going at all, as his sulking fits became more and more of a burden to me. The only thing that kept me going was the knowledge that I needed the break myself. I needed some space to do things that I needed to do, not just serving him or living in his back pocket, as it were. I needed room to breathe, and his constant possessiveness was beginning to smother me. I loved my husband dearly, but I still needed time for myself. Was that so wrong? However, even the knowledge that my own needs were also important was nonetheless tempered by the feelings of guilt that started to plague me over deserting him for that one afternoon on my own. I knew I shouldn't feel guilty, but it's hard to convince yourself when someone you love seems so vulnerable and upset by your actions.

He began to resent any time I was out of his sight, and at the same time became more and more possessive, and increasingly jealous of my time, resenting anything or anybody that kept me away from him. Even my talking on the phone would upset him, because then I wasn't giving him my undivided attention, which he seemed to demand, more and more. If I was outside gardening or shovelling snow (not at the same time, of course) and stopped to talk with a neighbour or someone on the street, he would come outside immediately, to see who I was talking to and to listen in on the conversation. Not that we were ever talking about anything important, but it was embarrassing nonetheless. The lady next door actually commented one day as to how jealous my husband was, as he'd always come running outside, even if I was just talking with her. Others were also starting to recognize his possessiveness. By that time I had retired from my job, feeling that Edwin needed to be cared for in a way that was not possible with my working all day away from home. However I was not prepared to accept the fact that anything was radically wrong with him, other than making allowances for advancing age. He was just feeling somewhat vulnerable, perhaps, realizing his limitations and becoming more dependent on me. Again, I felt that the situation was quite understandable and I didn't mind being needed—not at all! I just needed to learn how to balance his dependency—or so I convinced myself.

Edwin loved to travel and had already taken many trips by himself, but once I was retired we were able to go more often as a couple, and we enjoyed travelling together on several lovely excursions. During our travels we met a lot of wonderful new people and made some great friends. He admitted on several occasions to being overwhelmed by the kindness of our friends, and insisted that I was the one that attracted them. However, this was not a problem, as in most cases he basked in their friendship and accepted it as his due. At times though, he would become surly and argumentative and I would have to take him back to our room before he embarrassed himself (or me) altogether. Then I would have to listen to his tirade of complaints: about me, about the place, about the food, about our friends, or whatever.

I learned to exercise a lot of self-control during those times, but the fact that they were becoming more and more frequent worried me a great deal. What was happening to him? What was happening to us? Why was he doing this to me—to us? What happened to the sweet, caring man that I married? Why was his personality changing so radically? Even more to the point, how much longer could I handle this without blowing up or losing my patience with him? However, I continued to make excuses for him, feeling that the travelling was putting too much pressure on him, and resolved to make things as easy for him as possible, especially when away from home and familiar surroundings.

Our last foreign trip was to Greece in April, where we enjoyed a wonderful vacation and saw many marvellous and amazing historical sights. However, it was also during that journey that I came to face the realization that my husband could no longer handle foreign travel and its inherent frustrations. The people in our tour group with Senior Tours were absolutely wonderful and very supportive, but by then it was apparent that my husband had a problem and that he leaned on me a great deal. However, the others in our group were more than willing to offer their help and encouragement whenever it was needed, and throughout our travels I was overwhelmed by their kindness and consideration. Indeed, without the help and support of others in the group, I doubt if I would have been able to hold myself together during those weeks in Greece. In spite of the enjoyment of sight-seeing in such a beautiful country with its awe-inspiring legacy of history, it was a very difficult trip in terms of the responsibility and care of my husband, and I realized that I could no longer permit him to travel so far from home and all that was familiar to him. Thus I determined that in the future our only traveling would involve a visit to Florida, a place that I knew he loved especially because of the weather, and was more like our own country in terms of language and accommodations. As you can imagine, it was a tremendous relief to return to Canada and home after that last major excursion abroad.

Thus it was that our next journey would be to Florida for the winter at the end of that same year. Edwin was very excited about going and planned the trip with great anticipation, as he detested our cold and damp Ontario winters, and looked forward to spending four months in a comfortably warm climate.

We left early on a Sunday morning near the end of November, encountering relatively little traffic on the highway and making good time to the border. From there we drove through heavy rain and high winds as we battled a hurricane en-route, so we decided to keep on driving in order to put the bad weather behind us. Despite the rain it was a pleasant trip, and we enjoyed chatting as the miles and the hours passed. We couldn't wait to hit the warm weather, leaving the winter behind us altogether, and we talked of all the things we planned to do in Florida that winter.

Not wanting to encounter rush hour traffic when starting out the following morning, we decided to push on until we gained the other side of Cincinnati before stopping for the night. It was a long day and a long drive, but at last, having reached our goal for the day, we stopped at the first motel we saw that was readily accessible from the highway. Thus we settled down for a good night's rest...or so we thought!

Little did we realize what lay ahead—or how our lives were destined to change forever that fateful night!

The Big Ticket Item

CHAPTER 5

After being home in Canada for a week, I was very discouraged to realize that poor Edwin was no better off. I thought things would settle down once he was home again in familiar surroundings, but that was not the case. He still had to be shown where everything was, such as his razor, toothbrush, etc., but then he wouldn't remember where they had come from and would replace them in a different location each time. As it was, he kept using my toothbrush too, so every day I'd have to explain to him which one was his.

One morning I opened the bathroom door after my shower to find Edwin standing there, so I asked him if he wanted to use the bathroom.

"Why would I want to use it?" he replied.

I said, "Well, perhaps you need to go to the toilet, or wash your face, or put in your teeth."

He then agreed that he did need to use the toilet but started to go downstairs. I quickly redirected him, having to show him where the toilet was, as usual. Afterwards he called me to come and show him how to wash his face. (At least he knew enough to realize he needed it washed.) Following that, I had to show him where his teeth were kept. And so it went, day after day, hour after hour.

As it was, my entire day was taken up showing him where to find everything, time and again, helping him dress (It was always the fault of the clothing when he had difficulty dressing), and trying to teach him how to do the normal, everyday things that he'd always done, and which were needful to everyday living. As well, I was constantly searching for things he'd put away in strange places, or hidden because he'd become convinced that someone was trying to steal them.

Dressing was quite an interesting exercise and required some assistance on my part, but as long as he could manage it himself, more or less, I needed to let him do it, regardless of the outcome, or his creativity. Otherwise he'd forget how to do it completely. So what if a button was mismatched, or if he was wearing two shirts, or had put on his sweater inside out? The important thing was that for the most part he had done it himself. That was important to him too, especially in regard to his feelings of accomplishment and self worth. Of course, I'd have to put out clean clothes for him every day. Otherwise he'd wear the same thing day after day, totally unconcerned about hygiene or dirty laundry, and only reacting to comfort and familiarity.

If I left his old clothes out with the new ones, he'd put on all of them. (He was wearing layers long before layering was in fashion.)

Some days he would come out to the living room totally twisted up in his undershirt and it would take some time and expertise to extricate him from it. I would tease him, while helping to untangle him from the shirt, which he always took good-naturedly, and we would both laugh over his predicament, rather than my trying to remonstrate with him. At least he'd tried to do it himself. In time, of course, even dressing became totally impossible for him to manage, and I'd have to dress him completely myself. However, until that time I encouraged him to do as much as possible for himself, praising him for any accomplishments, no matter how small. At times it was pretty frustrating, watching him struggle to do seemingly simple things that I could have done in minutes, but I had to force myself not to interfere, as I didn't want him to become too dependent on me. This worked only until he'd get completely frustrated, in which case, of course, I'd have to step in. Otherwise he'd have let me do everything for him and not even try to do it himself, which would have been a big mistake on my part, as he needed to be encouraged to do as much as possible for himself, as long as he was able. It isn't possible to teach Alzheimer's patients anything new, so it's doubly important to reaffirm skills they already know. They forget too easily as it is, to allow them to "unlearn" basic skills, and I certainly didn't want to precipitate that condition in my husband.

After we'd barely finished a meal, he would swear he hadn't eaten (you'd have thought his stomach would know), and then he'd berate me for having eaten myself, without feeding him. It wouldn't help to make him another meal either, for then he would just say he wasn't hungry anymore because I'd made him wait too long. Believe me, I actually tried that. Anything to keep the peace! It was the same with his pills. After taking them he'd swear he'd never had them at all. Probably the only reason he even remembered about his pills was because he had been taking them for so many years and the habit was strongly ingrained.

By that time he had undergone several Doctor's appointments and tests, but so far they had only confirmed that he did indeed have dementia, which we already knew beyond any shadow of doubt; but they were still reluctant to put any other name to it. It seems that doctors are very hesitant these days to use the "A" word. I'm not sure why and can only hazard a guess as to their reasoning. Apparently there is no definitive test for Alzheimer's disease, except post-mortem, so it is diagnostically impossible to prove someone actually has it until *after* they've died. Therefore, most doctors are very hesitant to declare someone has Alzheimer's for fear of being proven wrong. However, Edwin had all the classic symptoms of the disease, and the multitude of tests they had done only proved he had nothing else. Sometimes I wondered if it was worth putting him through all those tests and examinations, but I did want to be sure I was doing the right thing for him. It's so difficult to know sometimes, what is best for one you love.

Before actually stating that Edwin was suffering from Alzheimer's disease, the neurologist who examined him also diagnosed him as definitely having dementia. He then went on to set up appointments with all the other specialists he wanted Edwin to see, in order to determine the cause and extent of the damage to his brain, as well as the type of dementia from which he was suffering. It was really a very stressful time for both of us. After the first assessment however, I knew the outcome of all the tests could not be good, no matter what, for the neurologist had told me unequivocally, that Edwin's condition was irreversible. At that time he suggested that I seriously consider placement, stating that Edwin could never be left alone, and that he was in no way capable of coping with the various aspects of life anymore. He then reiterated the fact that he should be admitted to a nursing home as soon as possible, as it would be too much for me to handle on my own.

I thanked the Doctor for his concern, but declared, adamantly, that I could never do what he suggested. I could never do that to my husband! Nevertheless, he insisted that I take the time to think about it. I finally agreed—just to think about it—knowing full well that the entire concept was unthinkable, at least for me. I found myself on the verge of tears all the time those days, but I tried to put on a good front and remain calm and upbeat for Edwin's sake.

According to the doctors, and the numerous books I'd read on the subject, all these medical tests were vital in properly diagnosing Alzheimer's disease. In other words, a complete medical assessment was critical, in order to rule out other factors or conditions which could be causing the dementia. Many of those other causes, unlike Alzheimer's, are actually reversible, so it's important to know, before it's too late, if there is a cure available. I only wish that had been the case for us, but at least we knew for sure now. Until that point I had still harboured hopes that he had something curable, rather than Alzheimer's for which there was no hope.

Even today the disease is still ultimately inexorable, but scientists are beginning to see pinpoints of light in the long, dark tunnel of Alzheimer's disease. These tiny glimmers emerge as faint rays of hope in the struggle against dementia, as new drugs are being created that now can delay the onset of the disease, helping to alleviate some of the devastating symptoms for a time at least. Perhaps tomorrow will see even more enlightenment! We can only hope!

It was Wednesday, the 10th of April, just thirteen days after we'd left Florida. When I asked Edwin what day it was, he replied, "Sunday."

Then I asked him what month it was, and he answered, "December."

Next I asked for the year.

"I don't know," he replied. "It's 1970 something."

Obviously he still had no concept of time. Unfortunately, that is one of the standard problems with Alzheimer's patients: their total lack of any sense regarding time, including months, days, or even the year. One specialist, in asking him these same questions, became very impatient with him, almost acting as though he believed he was doing it on purpose, or simply not trying. Poor Edwin just became more and more flustered and unnerved, causing me to become rather upset with the doctor myself. I was still constantly having to remind myself that Edwin was not responsible, that he really didn't know what he was doing, and that it was equally frustrating for him. I should think a doctor would understand this all too well, but apparently not. It does make me appreciate doctors who *are* kind and patient all the more though. In cases such as these, bedside manner really can be important. I don't care how clever a doctor is, antagonizing or upsetting the patient would seem to be counter-productive to me. I worked hard to maintain an aura of peace for my husband, who was volatile at best, and I didn't need any medical professional, who should have known better, upsetting him unnecessarily!

Incidentally, that particular day was our wedding anniversary, whether Edwin realized it or not; so I took my husband out for dinner that night, along with Pat and Bill, a lovely young couple, neighbours of ours, who had looked after the house for us while we were away in Florida. Thus it was an anniversary celebration, as well as a way of thanking them for their help. It turned out to be quite an enjoyable evening, and Edwin seemed to enjoy the outing as well, although he ate very little of his dinner and I brought most of it home. I think the restaurant setting was a bit overwhelming for him, but he did enjoy the company, and he ate the rest of his meal the following day at home.

While at the restaurant we ran into a mutual friend who later mentioned to Pat and Bill that he was surprised at the change in my husband. He commented especially on the fact that Edwin's eyes looked vacant, and he was shocked and saddened, having last seen us just that past summer, at which time he'd enjoyed a delightful conversation with him. Thus, the change he saw in him was quite startling.

Shortly after that our family doctor also began to agree with the specialist that something needed to be done about Edwin, strongly recommending the need for me to put him into a nursing home. Of course I was just as adamant in refusing. How could I possibly do that to my husband? I'd married him "for better or worse," and I meant to stick by my vows. He needed me and I didn't plan to desert him. The doctor then contacted my husband's son, to try and get him to talk some sense into me, but he agreed with my decision to keep him at home and that was final. However, having heard from the doctor personally, seemed to bring the fact of his father's condition home more forcefully to his son than before, and he became quite concerned about his dad, so much so that he informed me of his intention to visit more often. Needless to say, I was pleased to hear it, and encouraged him to do so, as often as he wished. Of course Edwin wasn't so sure about it. He didn't want company in the house, no matter who it was, and was quite vocal on the subject. At that point he had become quite territorial and didn't want anyone invading his privacy. However, I'm convinced that he did enjoy his son's visits while he was there, even if he wouldn't admit it.

Strangely enough, though he was very protective about his home, Edwin had no actual knowledge of having owned the house for 39 years, much less having lived there all that time. He was convinced we were just renting the place, since it was all new to him and seemingly not familiar in any way. Thus he was always complaining about the things he planned to tell the landlord, who, incidentally, he was certain was "ripping us off." Nothing would convince him otherwise, so I just had to let it go. You couldn't argue with him, as he *knew* he was right, so I just had to go along with him in whatever he said or believed, or at least use it to advantage in learning to keep him under control—albeit not an easy undertaking at best. As long as what he believed, or what he wanted to do, wasn't detrimental to him or his health, I would agree with him or do it with him, just to keep him calm and content. It made things a lot easier to cope with in the end, and saved the arguments for situations which required my resistance.

One of the doctors I had taken him to see at the insistence of his neurologist, was a specialist in geriatric medicine and more specifically in problems of dementia. The gerontologist conducted some experimental tests with Edwin, not unlike some of the tests I had tried myself in Florida, in order to ascertain the extent of his dementia. In one of them he instructed him to draw a circle, which he managed to do with not too much difficulty. Then he was asked to draw the face of a clock in that circle. Edwin started with 12 at the top of the circle and I was encouraged, thinking he would do it correctly. However, he then proceeded to add the numbers, in the correct order, except that the 12 now became part of the 1, 2, 3, 4 series, all along the right side of the circle, ending with 12 at the bottom. Next he was asked to draw three o'clock, for which he drew one arrow pointing to the three. So much for telling time! He had the numbers and the sequence right but not the placement, and he was missing the second hand of the clock. Apparently this is a very revealing test.

Another test the doctor conducted was to quote a well-known saying and have Edwin supply the last few words. One of them was a very well known proverb: "People who live in glass houses...." Edwin supplied the missing words, "shouldn't throw stones." (This was the only one he was able to answer.) However, when asked to define the meaning of this quotation, it lost something in his translation.

He replied, "If you live in a glass house, you shouldn't throw things or you'll smash the glass."

The basic idea was correct but the original concept was lost. In other words, he was still able to understand some things, realistically, but was unable to think in abstracts.

Simple math and memory tests were also administered, but with less than satisfactory results, at least in my estimation, as he failed miserably. The math problems were very basic but totally beyond Edwin's expertise, somewhat surprising for one who had excelled at math and related electronics in the past. (Many specialists in the medical field are claiming now that these same math tests are more effective in satisfying the diagnosis of Alzheimer's disease than all the medical tests the patients must undergo.)

I have to admit though, that if those tests had been scored by time, even I would have had trouble with one of them. Arithmetic was never my forte and counting backwards by sevens from 100 is not the easiest thing to do, at least not quickly. In this case, however, speed is not an important factor, just the ability to think it through.

Another test involved a list of 15 words, requiring the patient to see how many he could recall a short time later. As it was, Edwin completely forgot there was a list, so he had nothing to recall. A similar test involved only four words to be recalled later but the results were the same. In other words, Edwin's short-term memory was gone, totally. The only thing remaining for him was his long ago past, but as time evolved, it too faded away into a cloud of mist.

Other tests had much the same results, not surprisingly, and the doctor then went on to give him a thorough physical examination. Following that, he put Edwin into another room while he talked with me.

Sitting down beside me, he said very seriously, "This is not good! In fact, this is very bad! Your husband has severe dementia and I strongly suspect Alzheimer's."

He then asked me what my investment was in this situation?

I wasn't certain exactly what he meant but I replied, "He's my husband, for better or for worse, and I love him. What else can I say?"

He then went on to say that most couples had a lifetime of 30 or 40 years together, so they had their memories, but since our time together had been relatively short, only a few years, it was an entirely different situation, at least according to him.

"I'm afraid you've bought the 'big ticket item,' and I wouldn't blame you for jumping ship," he said. "You're still young and attractive, and I'd strongly recommend your walking away from this while you can."

I was shocked at his attitude! Of course I declined, reiterating "for better or worse," but I realized then that I was in for the long haul, no matter what, since I knew in my heart that there was no way I could walk out on my husband now. I was, however, very disappointed and disillusioned by the doctor's suggestion that I did have another option. I honestly did not feel that I had any other alternative and was appalled by his apparent callousness. I realize he was only trying to think of my welfare, but nevertheless, life has no guarantees and one has to take the good with the bad, no matter how bad, and my life was no exception.

After that appointment, Edwin was convinced that the doctor was "after me," and accused him of "devouring me with his eyes." He maintained that the doctor couldn't keep his eyes off me, and nothing I said could convince him otherwise. Of course the doctor did keep looking at me, but in truth it was to gauge my reaction, as well as for confirmation of the facts as related by my husband in answer to his questions. Apart from being jealous, however, it also pleased Edwin to think that someone else was interested in his wife. He was actually quite proud to think that he "owned" a wife that other men desired. He was so delighted about that aspect of it that I gave up trying to argue with him. If it made him happy to think that way, then I could live with it. As it was, he had become increasingly jealous by that time of anyone I talked to, man or woman, and anything that took up my time, including walking, reading or studying, gardening, shovelling snow, or even watching TV instead of going to bed. He wanted me with him, and attending to him, 24 hours a day, and it had become an obsession with him, as he declared on numerous occasions that "such was the duty of a wife." In actuality it was becoming impossible to leave him alone at all any more, as I feared for his safety, so in essence he was getting his wish, even as I was growing more and more exhausted and run down.

When the doctor asked Edwin if he had any children, he promptly replied "No."

I corrected him of course, telling the doctor about his son. However, then I began to see things from his perspective. Maybe he was thinking only in terms of children being young, in which case he had no young kids. Before discounting everything he would say, I had to consider where he was coming from, realizing that he could no longer think in abstracts, but only understood words at face value. This new insight helped me to understand him a lot better after that, though unfortunately, not always.

Along with the Alzheimer's Edwin had also developed a habit of speaking his mind, whatever that might be, and saying anything that came into his head, without considering the consequences. No longer constrained by social mores, he lacked the insight he once possessed in knowing when to speak and when to refrain. Now there were no restraints and he said what he thought, which could be very embarrassing at times. One of those incidents involved our next visit to that same doctor. By then, Edwin had already forgotten who he was or what he looked like. As we waited in the reception area for our one o'clock appointment, the doctor returned from lunch, walking right past us to enter his own office. I was mortified to hear Edwin speaking out loud, as the doctor walked past.

He asked, "Who is that big, fat 'lunk' anyway?"

I tried to hush him, explaining that it was the doctor himself, but he didn't remember ever having seen him before.

Just one of life's embarrassing moments!

Time and No Time Again

Time to myself was very precious and rare those days, and as the disease progressed, such occasions became fewer and farther between. When my husband was sleeping or sitting in a chair dozing, I would try to take advantage of the break by sitting down for a while myself, perhaps with a good book, or using the time to catch up on some unfinished task, or attempting to do so at any rate. Those breaks were short and sweet and although not terribly satisfactory, they still helped to temper the strain of constantly dancing attendance to Edwin and his needs. Most often though, he was continually underfoot and begging for attention. Actually, at times I would trip over him, he would be so close to me, and it was very difficult to accomplish anything with him around. Vacuuming was the worst, as he was always right behind me when I'd try to back up. Even to answer the call of nature was a trial, as the minute I'd enclose myself in the bathroom he'd start calling for me. I would always tell him where I was going, and he'd see me enter the door, but within minutes he would have forgotten where I'd gone. I'd try answering his calls too, but he could never seem to ascertain where my voice was coming from and he'd move away from the door to look for me. If I flushed the toilet or ran the water, he'd hear it running down the pipes into the basement and think I was down there. Since the basement was usually dark, he would be afraid to go down there looking for me, but on emerging from the bathroom I'd often find him sitting halfway down the stairs, peering into the dark, convinced I was down there and waiting for me to come back upstairs. My worst nightmare was to imagine him some day tumbling down those steep stairs, so I desperately tried to keep him away from that area as much as possible. He'd already survived a number of bad falls by that time and I certainly didn't want to take any chances.

One day we were sitting on the patio, enjoying the lovely weather and a cup of tea. Not yet incontinent at that point, Edwin announced his intention of going to the bathroom and went back inside. When he hadn't returned some time later, I became concerned and went looking for him. I found him in the bedroom lying down and pouting. He was in a foul mood and railed at me for having left him all alone. He demanded to know where I had gone and why I had left him. Of course, I wasn't the one who had left, but how could I explain that to him? The inability of those with Alzheimer's to comprehend or process knowledge can be extremely frustrating to the caregiver, who is wrongfully accused of all manner of sins, both of commission and omission, but until I understood that facet of the disease, I suffered agonies of frustration, and humiliation, and even guilt.

As mentioned in a previous chapter, many times Edwin would ask me if I'd had dinner yet, and when I'd reply in the affirmative, he'd become angry at me for having fed myself and not him. No amount of arguing would convince him otherwise, even though he had just finished a lovely dinner. At times I'd be tempted to wonder if it was worth the effort even trying to make things nice for him, but in my heart I knew the only possible answer was yes. Even though he couldn't remember things that happened, sometimes only moments before, I knew that I had given him satisfaction for that moment in time. That alone was my reward, knowing I was doing my best to give him quality of life, even if it did lack quantity, at least in time and memory for him.

The only part of the day I could practically guarantee having time to myself was early in the morning, as Edwin had usually worn himself out by then, having wandered about the house most of the night. However, I was usually worn out by then too, simply from trying to keep up with him. He didn't just walk either, although at times he merely paced back and forth, moving with purpose, yet going nowhere.

Other times he was quite industrious, wrapping things in Kleenex or toilet paper (he wasn't choosy), including his six-hundred-dollar hearing aid, which ultimately got thrown out in the garbage along with the rest of his dirty Kleenex while he was in the hospital. He was always secreting things away as well, hiding them in the most unlikely places, so almost every day we had a "search party" looking for the things he had hidden, before we could go anywhere or even get him properly dressed. Actually he was quite ingenious in his hiding places and always coming up with new ones. It was quite a challenge! In fact, at times he was so clever it was hard to believe he really didn't know what he was doing. Through all of this: the search and rescue, the accusations, the frustrating argumentativeness, and the abject deviousness, I was forced, constantly, to remind myself that he wasn't responsible, that he really didn't know what he was doing; but sometimes it was hard to convince myself. Some of the things he did seemed so premeditated, so devious, it was hard to realize it wasn't planned by a clever, conniving brain.

Actually, when you think of it, a lot of his activities reflected the way a very young child would behave, and children, certainly, are not responsible. There is one subtle difference, however. A child can learn! Someone with Alzheimer's cannot learn anything new, which is why it is so important that we help them by reaffirming what they already know, such as how to feed or dress themselves, until even that becomes an impossibility. As it was, in Edwin's case, it was becoming increasingly difficult to give him any task to do, no matter how small, as he just couldn't seem to understand the directions any more. In some ways it was worse that having a young child because, as mentioned before, a child can learn. Also, when children misbehave we can punish them, (appropriately, of course) so they won't repeat their actions, but I certainly could not punish Edwin, as he had no idea what he was doing wrong.

Dressing was also becoming more difficult for him and some days he just refused to dress at all. He'd stay in his pyjamas all day (most unusual for him), but if it wasn't necessary to go out for any reason, I'd just let it ride, rather than facing the struggle of trying to get him dressed. Whenever possible, it was a lot easier—on both of us—just to let him have his own way. I was tired of struggling with him, and perhaps he was weary of it all as well. Who knows? I do know that it was becoming more and more difficult for him to dress himself and maybe some days he just lacked the energy to do so.

One evening we were sitting companionably in the TV room when Edwin suddenly stood up and walked into the bedroom. When he returned he was wearing only his undershirt, shoes, and socks—nothing more! He proceeded, quite nonchalantly, to sit down beside me again and watch the television.

"Aren't you going to put on your pyjamas?" I asked, discreetly.

"You mean I don't have them on?" he replied, looking very surprised indeed.

One day, after taking him to the doctor's office, I suddenly realized that his shirt was buttoned up incorrectly. By the time I noticed, it was too late, so I said nothing. However, the doctor noticed it and commented on it. Poor Edwin had no idea what he was talking about, so the doctor pointed out the left-over button at the top of his shirt.

Edwin's reply was to ask, "Why, is that button any better than the rest?"

The doctor just gave up in disgust. (Yes, I said disgust!) I soon discovered, to my dismay, that not all doctors had the aptitude or the patience to deal with situations of this nature. Yet, as a caregiver, I had no choice. I had to learn, or lose! No one chooses to be put into this situation, but it happens, and it can happen to anyone—even the President of the United States! No one is immune! The sooner we come to realize this, I firmly believe, the sooner we will start reaching out to others going through similar experiences. Only then shall we be able to deal with it more humanely, accepting Alzheimer's disease, and other related forms of dementia, as a fact of life, instead of something to be ashamed of, something to hide in the closet as it were.

In a way it was good that the doctor was able to see first-hand what I was experiencing every day, even though it was only a very small example of what we put up with every day and all day long. Sometimes, I think they really don't have any idea what we're going through, so they don't know how to help. After that appointment, the doctor seemed to become far more understanding and helpful, and even offered to fill out a form for us, enabling me to acquire a Handicapped Parking sticker, an item which proved to be a great help, since Edwin had to go everywhere with me but had difficulty walking any distance.

Sometimes Edwin would be convinced he could hear the phone ringing and ringing, and he'd wonder why I wouldn't answer it. (His ears must have been ringing because it certainly wasn't the phone!) He would then demand to know who was calling me that I didn't want him to know about, having convinced himself that this was the reason I wouldn't answer the phone. Thinking to forestall his tirade, on occasion I'd try pretending to answer the phone when he'd think he heard it ringing. However, then he'd demand to know who was calling, and would accuse me of lying if I said no one, or that it was a wrong number. Those were definitely "no win" situations!

At other times when the phone actually was ringing and I'd answer it, he'd start yelling and swearing at me because I was ignoring him by answering the phone. He never used to swear before, and it would be very embarrassing when the person on the phone was able to hear him. In fact, in most cases they were shocked to think that he could do something like that, having known him before his illness. (Even I was shocked at times!) Needless to say, it could be very stressful, so I stayed off the phone as much as possible.

Another thing about the telephone was that whenever it did ring, Edwin would turn off the television in order to listen in on my conversation. He was unable to operate the remote control any more but he would march up to the TV and hit the Off button. Then he'd hang over my shoulder, or skulk by the door of my room, to hear what I was saying. In fact, if he could find another phone, he'd pick it up to hear both sides of the conversation. When I'd ask him to hang up the phone he'd refuse.

"It's my phone!" he would state, unequivocally. "I can use it whenever I want!"

In the end I finally had to give up trying to stop him from listening in, but it was disconcerting, never being able to have a private conversation with anyone. I was beginning to feel cut off from the world, in more ways than one!

I took Edwin out for a tea party at Alma's one day, along with his son and daughter-in-law and the grandchildren. We had a nice visit and Edwin behaved himself quite well, sitting quietly and enjoying his food. However, when we put on our coats to leave, he remained seated in Alma's comfortable chair.

I went over to him and said, "Would you like to go home now?"

He answered meekly, "Yes, please."

In so many ways he was like a child again, very tractable at times, but also given to temper tantrums and wanting his own way. The trouble was I never knew which one to expect!

Edwin had always used handkerchiefs and those days were no exception, especially since he had developed a penchant for eating Kleenex, not to mention using up an entire box in one sitting, just to wrap his belongings. However, even with the handkerchiefs I'd have to keep my eye on him to make sure he didn't throw them out in the garbage, along with whatever else he'd decided to wrap inside them. One night, before I could stop him, he stuffed his handkerchief into his dish of chicken-pot-pie. What a mess! I asked him, gently, not to do it again, but he had no concept of what he'd done wrong.

As the disease progressed he started wrapping more things in his handkerchiefs, gross things, such as when he went to the toilet. Sometimes it was very difficult, having to clean up after him, and at times it was just easier to throw the entire "package" away.

One night there was a thunderstorm and poor Edwin was terrified. That was most unusual for him, since storms never used to bother him. In fact, he always used to laugh at me when I was nervous during a storm.

Our roles were steadily reversing!

Every day, by then, was a new beginning for Edwin, like starting out with a clean slate. He had no past, no memories, just the here and now. Each day he would have to ask me where his clothes were, what he should wear, where his wallet was, where his keys were, and so on. At bedtime he'd suddenly decide to explore the place where we were staying that night, and he could never understand why we were the only ones staying there.

"Surely there must be other people needing a shelter," he'd say to me.

"No," I'd assure him, "we're the only ones here."

"Where are the others? Where did everybody go?"

"There are no others," I'd tell him again and again.

Then he'd ask, "Where did we stay last night?"

Some evenings he would go on and on about how expensive it was to stay in places like this, referring to our home, which at other times he'd think we were renting. On those occasions he'd also begin a litany of complaints about things he intended to tell the landlord who, incidentally, he was still convinced, was ripping us off.

As time went on, I began to notice that Edwin was experiencing greater difficulty in locating the words he wanted to use. He'd know what he was talking about but just couldn't find the right word for it. One night he tried to ask me about how I had cooked the dinner. Not being able to remember the word for stove, he became very excited and finally yelled out, "You know...Fire! Fire!...Hot! Hot!"

At times he could be quite ingenious at choosing alternative words for those he couldn't remember. Thank goodness for his extensive vocabulary to begin with, as that helped him greatly in expressing himself those days. When he couldn't remember the word for his zipper he called it a "slide." When he talked one day about hoping to win the "cross-word-puzzle" he was actually referring to the "Lotto 649," but couldn't think of the right name for it.

On the whole, I think that one of the reasons he was able to appear so normal at times, at least in public, was due to his language skills. His vocabulary had always been far superior to the average person (inherently British, I suspect), so even with the loss of some words, he still had a fairly normal range.

I continued trying to get Edwin to help with chores, just to keep him active and involved, but it was becoming more difficult and I had to keep a close eye on him. When I'd get his help clearing the table, he'd just as readily carry the items past the kitchen, to his bedroom or wherever his fancy took him at the time. It was nothing for me to find the mustard or mayonnaise in his bedroom, alongside his underwear, or even one of his slippers in the fridge, beside the carton of milk. When my napkin ring disappeared one day, he swore he'd had nothing to do with it, but it finally turned up in the fridge, wrapped around the end of a loaf of bread!

One of his daily chores was to turn down the bed covers before going to bed each night, although I still had to remind him every time, and even then he wouldn't always do it. One evening I discovered that he had turned down the covers on his side of the bed correctly, but my side had been turned up, from the bottom! (Maybe he was trying to tell me something!) Strangely enough, he had no idea that it wasn't done properly, and was actually quite pleased with his efforts, convinced that he had done a good job.

We were late getting home one evening, as I'd had a number of errands to run. Since Edwin was hungry,

I decided to take him to his favourite restaurant, the Red Lobster, where he thoroughly enjoyed a meal of Shrimp Fettuccine, and was quite content with the world. However, barely an hour after returning home, he asked me what we were having for dinner. I couldn't believe it! I was still feeling very full from our lovely meal and here he was asking about food again.

"We already had dinner," I told him.

"No we didn't!" he exclaimed.

"Yes we did!" I said. "We ate at the Red Lobster."

"Well," he said. "If that was lobster, that's the smallest damn lobster I've ever seen!"

I started to laugh and couldn't stop. In my imagination, I kept picturing our shrimp as tiny lobsters, and I laughed until I cried. In fact, I laughed so hard, Edwin began laughing too, even though he had no idea what we were laughing about. He still loved a good joke!

One night he went on and on about some papers that we were supposed to sign. I didn't have a clue what he was talking about, unfortunately, which only made him more upset. I tried to calm him down but without success. Finally, in total disgust, he went into the bedroom and slammed the door. At such times he'd usually go to bed so I found it best just to leave him alone. The next day, sure enough, he'd forgotten all about it. However, that evening he started in again, on the same subject. In most cases he would forget entirely, but there were times when he would bring up the same subject night after night, and this was one of them. After a while I'd find it very difficult just to keep my cool, let alone try to help him. In that instance he accused me of trying to make him 'think he was crazy, when he's not!' Unfortunately, I just did not know all the answers.

It finally came to the point that I realized it was no longer possible to have a meaningful conversation with my husband any more. If we were speaking about a particular person, he'd ask, "Who's that?" Then, by the time I'd have explained who they were, he'd have forgotten what we were talking about! If I'd mention something we'd just seen on TV, he would have forgotten about it already, just seconds after having seen it. For example, one night there was a picture of a lawn mower cutting a large, beautiful, green lawn on TV, and I commented on the lovely lawn.

"What lawn?" Edwin asked.

I said, "That one," pointing to the TV set.

He said, "Which one?"

I replied, "The one on the television!"

By the time he looked back at the TV again, the lawn was no longer there, of course, so then he went on and on about my imagining things! That same scenario would be repeated over and over until it would drive me crazy. However, if I refused to answer his questions any more, he'd get very annoyed as well. I just couldn't win!

Speaking of lawns, gardening was another passion that helped me to keep my sanity, during those long, lonely months with Edwin. Of course I thought I was creating a beautiful garden for my future use as well, but unfortunately that wasn't to be, as ultimately, I had to give up the house and move to an apartment building. (It costs a lot of money to keep someone in a nursing home and eventually our budget just couldn't handle it anymore, since it was costing me more per month for Edwin than it did for myself.) However, I'm grateful for the cathartic value of the hard work I put into my garden, and the time I was able to invest in such endeavours. I would bring my husband outside, to sit among the beautiful flowers while I worked, allowing him to enjoy the beauty of the garden and the fresh air; while at the same time he could see me and know I was still there for him. As well, I'd talk to him regularly, which he also found comforting and reassuring, so he was content to sit in his comfortable chair until I came to take him back inside. One day he even told me that he thought there were three woman living in our house: one that did the gardening, one that did the cooking, and the third one who drove him in the car to all his appointments. He couldn't grasp the fact that we were all one person. Mind you, at that point I think I felt like more than one person too. Having to do everything for someone, and being on call, as it were, for 24 hours a day, stretches a person to the limits of their endurance.

Walking was another great exercise, which helped me stay sane. I was still taking advantage of those early morning hours, while Edwin was still sleeping, and would rise at 5 a.m. to go for a 7-kilometer walk, before coming home to prepare his breakfast. That exercise was my salvation—my sanity—and I valued the time immensely. I could usually guarantee his sleeping at least until 7:00 a.m., but often 8:00 or 9:00. However, just to be on the safe side, I continued to use the two-way radios I'd purchased in Florida, which could cover quite a fair distance. I'd wear one on my belt, with an ear phone in my ear, and set the other one on transmit so I could hear immediately if my husband did happen to get up earlier. These proved very effective, and any time I did hear him stirring I'd head straight for home. (Only once did I not get home fast enough, and he met me halfway up the street wearing only his underwear!)

The radios even allowed me to stop off at a neighbour's house for a quick coffee some mornings, when I desperately needed someone to talk to. My dear friend Alma, who lived just up the street from us, always had a ready ear to listen and a soft shoulder to cry on, and when I could no longer bear the burden alone, she was always there for me. How I thank God for bringing her into my life! She was a real blessing to me and helped me through many a difficult time, when I'd think I just couldn't go on any longer. She helped me by sharing my burden and I will always be grateful to her, and to my friends Pat and Bill, another wonderful couple that I'm sure the Lord brought into my life for that purpose. It was the time spent with these special friends that gave me the strength and the courage to carry on. We all need some human support at one time or another, to keep us from going over the edge, and they were mine. I shall always be grateful to everyone that gave me help and encouragement during those difficult days, but for those three special people most of all.

Never discount the value of true friendship. Had it not been for the many friends I met along the way—some long-time pals, others in passing—I doubt I could have withstood all the trials and tribulations I faced during those long, dark years. I truly believe that each one came into my life for a reason, if only for a season, and I continue to thank God for every one of them, time and again.

Where the Hat Is

Getting ready for bed one night, Edwin asked me where the doctor was, saying he wanted his pills. I told him that I would give him his pill. Then he asked me why I would give it to him instead of the doctor, and was it because the doctor had already gone to bed? I don't know where he thought we were living at that time, but certainly not in our own private house. Later on he asked me if I was going to send him home. I tried to explain that we were already in our own home, but he couldn't seem to grasp it. He was so afraid of losing me, but I would never have left him. I only wished that I knew how to make him understand that fact.

There were times, however, when he realized quite clearly our ownership of the house, at least during his first year with the disease. In fact it almost seemed a burden to him and he would worry about my ability to cope because of his increasing inability to help. At those times he would insist that it was time to sell the house and simplify our living arrangements. I was finally beginning to agree with him, having nightmares myself about the times he would be confused and disorientated; terrified of his falling down the basement stairs, or something equally horrific. I was able to see the wisdom in such a decision, realizing it was best to let the house go, while he was still able to make decisions for himself, at least during his more lucid periods. Also, I realized all too clearly that there was no way I could look after the place myself, and do all the necessary repairs, not to mention the upkeep and taxes. Thus I started to consider his proposal, seriously weighing the pros and cons of the situation.

Actually, Edwin had wanted to sell the house three years before, with the idea of buying a small condo we could then close up, while spending the winters in Florida, or even Spain. Originally, he had planned to sell the house and move to Spain but I soon talked him out of that idea, realizing it was sheer folly to consider such a move at our age. However, the plan to spend only the winters in Florida seemed more reasonable and I was willing to consider it. Even then, though, I had sensed his need to be surrounded by familiar things and balked at the idea at first. In fact, when we travelled, as we'd done frequently in the past, I tried whenever possible to unpack his things and place them in the same location they would be in at home. It made things less stressful for him, thus making the travel more enjoyable for both of us. By that time, however, nothing about the house was familiar to him any more, so it would not be a great hardship for him to part with the place. I had come to love our home myself as well, especially the garden, which was so cathartic for me, but as I became more and more involved with Edwin's daily needs, I had less and less time to give to the house. Perhaps it was time to consider moving to a condo.

I should reiterate at this juncture that Edwin did have times—even hours—of complete lucidity, when he made perfect sense, and we could enjoy interesting conversations and illuminating discussions. Evenings and nights for him were never good, but often during the day he could be relatively normal for a few hours. I say relatively, as he'd still have his problems, but at those times he would be cognizant of them, aware of his inability to remember things and conscious of his frustrations. However, during those times when he was completely lucid, he would still continue to insist on my remaining with him, and I think, even then, he was afraid to be alone, lest he sink once more into his debilitating fog.

It was during one of those periods that we discussed selling the house. Even though he recognized the necessity of selling it, realizing he was no longer able to maintain it, he was still not at home in the house himself any more. In other words, he was totally coherent and could reasonably discuss a situation, as in the case of selling the house, but he still had areas that were completely lost to him, such as memories of having lived in the house for the last 39 years. It would almost seem like a contradiction in terms, but let me assure you, it is possible. Compare it, if you will, to someone who has lost a leg or an arm. They could never re-grow the missing limb, but they are no less a person without it. They can still think and function, except in areas requiring the use of that missing part. So too, a person suffering from dementia can still have periods of complete lucidity. The damaged area of their brain is gone for good—it can't grow again either—but the rest of the brain can function quite well, at least during the earlier stages of the disease. As it advances, however, those periods of lucidity become fewer and farther between until they are finally lost forever.

Once Edwin had made up his mind to sell the house there was no stopping him. I had warned him to think it over carefully as it would be a big move for us, but he was determined to do it as soon as possible. Since the house no longer held any real ties for him, I could see that it might be a good move, especially for him, and it would certainly relieve our financial burdens, which were beginning to concern me. I realized as well though, that I would greatly miss the place myself, especially the garden, where I had been able to work out a lot of my frustrations. It had become such a beautiful spot too, with flowers and pathways and all the added touches I had so lovingly created, and we'd enjoyed sitting out there together during the good weather in summer and long into the autumn. I would sorely miss those times.

I asked him where we would live if we sold the house, and did he have anything in mind? He just said that he didn't know, but he would trust me to find something. I was flattered by his trust in me, but at the same time I didn't want to make any decisions by myself. I agreed with his previous suggestion in regard to a condo, stating the obvious, that at least there would be no snow to shovel, and no grass to cut, and we could just lock the door when we went away, with no worries about thieves breaking in. He actually became very excited about the prospect and talked of nothing else for several weeks. Since he didn't know his own home any more, I realized it really didn't matter to him where he lived, but I still found it all very sad. At any rate, we listed the house, and Edwin himself signed all the papers, so he was still very much involved in the transaction.

When updating his son on his father's condition I also gave him the news about selling the house. He was shocked and troubled about our decision—understandably so—but I realized now that it had to be done, and the sooner the better, while Edwin could still be a part of the process. Neither of us were able to look after the house properly any more, and if Edwin eventually ended up in a nursing home (God forbid!), then I wouldn't be able to afford the upkeep anyway. Unfortunately his son accused me of pushing the deal through myself, stating that his father swore he'd never sell his house, and I could understand where he was coming from. Probably his father did feel that way in the past, but the past was gone, and we had to face the future—an uncertain future at best. I tried to explain to him that it really was his father's idea to sell the house, but that I was forced to agree, given the circumstances. However, I really don't think his son was able to grasp the fact that the house no longer bore any ties for his father; that it had become completely strange to him. I found it hard enough, myself, to comprehend, especially after he'd lived there for more than 39 years now. Even for me, after living with the results of this deadly disease for several months, it was still unthinkable and almost unbelievable! However, it was all too true unfortunately, even though I'd have given anything to reverse the situation—everything I owned—just to make it not be true!

At any rate, we finally went ahead and listed the house—a very sad day for me—but it really was for the best, as time certainly proved. Edwin had no problem whatever when it came time to sign the papers, and the house finally sold, but I had a hard time signing them myself. I kept thinking it couldn't be happening! I just wanted to tear up the contract; tell them it was a mistake; anything but go through with it, but in the end I realized it had to be done. I had no other choice. It had taken almost two months to sell and during that time we spent many hours looking for a nice condo, where Edwin could feel at home and daily living would become more manageable, for both of us. Unfortunately, as it turned out, my husband never did get to live in the new place, and it was a sad move for me, alone again—but that's another story, another day!

While we continued to live in our home, more and more the place became strange and unfamiliar to Edwin, and I realized afresh the validity of our decision.

That house meant nothing to him any more. In fact, as time passed, it seemed to be a focal point of his continuing confusion. Eventually he came to be living in a different location almost daily. I must say as well, that he never lacked for variety in his imaginative ventures. Our home venue changed regularly every evening, from a rented house, to a luxury hotel, a boarding school in England, a hospital (also in England), a dentist's office, a nursing home, a guest house, and almost any other setting you could imagine. As well, our location would change between Florida, Canada and England, although towards the end it settled mainly in London, England. (Well, it certainly was a cheap way to travel!)

My role constantly changed as well, covering the gamut from gardener, to cook, nurse, doctor, driver, caretaker, "the boy," school mistress, and even "Sally Ann." (Talk about a split personality! Mine was fractured!)

When he began referring to me as the person running the boarding school where he lived, I would try reminding him that I was his wife and nothing else. He would look genuinely shocked at that revelation, unable to take it in. Then, five minutes later he'd be back at the boarding school again, so I'd finally give up trying. One evening, however, after being in the school all day, at least in his own mind, he turned to me, earnestly seeking an answer to his question.

"Seriously now, do you have any idea where my wife is?"

Sometimes I just didn't know what to say any more. He simply wouldn't—or couldn't—accept the truth, so there was no point really in trying to explain. I'd try to appease him, as suggested in the many books I'd read on the subject, by asking him to tell me about his wife, encouraging him to talk about her, and thereby diverting him from his original contention. He'd then give me a wonderfully flattering description of myself, so I'd know it really was me he was searching for. Unfortunately, he just didn't recognize my face anymore. By then, I existed only in his mind, a paragon of virtue, something between Florence Nightingale and an angel! If only it were true! However, too well I knew my own shortcomings when it came to dealing with the fears and frustrations of living daily with such a devastating disease. I was no angel! Believe me, I was just as human as anyone else, an ordinary person, thrust suddenly and sadly into an extraordinary situation from which there was no escape and no reprieve.

Another evening, another torrent of questions, but still there was no acceptance of the truth. First he went on about wanting to take a tour of his "new home." After over 39 years it was still *new* to him! Again, he was convinced that we were living in London, England.

"How can we afford this place? Are there no other tenants? Why not? Is it too expensive, or what?"

As if those questions weren't enough, after that he continued on a different line of queries.

"How did we get all the furniture here? Did any get damaged? How long have you lived here? How did you come across this place? Was it advertised, a paper ad?"

The questions just didn't stop and he'd ask the

same ones over and over, relentlessly going on, until I'd feel like screaming myself, "Stop! Stop! Stop!" I would try to answer him, even making up the answers if it would help, but to no avail. It would just go on and on, endlessly!

A few days later we went over to his son's house for their daughter's second birthday. While there, Edwin shocked everyone by proceeding to tell anyone who would listen all about the house he had inherited from his father and mother, just a few doors away from where I lived. He also told them that the new house had all the same furniture and pictures in it as his house. He couldn't understand why no one seemed particularly excited about it, or even interested in his story. I think for the most part they were embarrassed for him. They kept looking at me for verification, but I'd just shake my head, indicating there was no truth to his story, so they just looked the other way, making no response to him; not really knowing just what to say in the circumstances.

That same evening I was just performing the last minute chores before retiring for the night, making sure the doors were locked and the alarm engaged, turning down the thermostat, and shutting off the lights. All the usual tasks one does before going to bed.

Edwin was already in bed, when he called for me to come. "I have a question for you," he said. "Is there some sort of electrical device in the bed pillows?"

"No, of course not," I answered him. "Why do you ask?"

"Because," he replied, "whenever I turned my pillow over, it beeped."

I assured him there was no such thing, but I had to smile. He must have heard me setting the thermostat for the night!

One day Edwin asked me to get a thousand dollars out of the bank for him. I was surprised at his request so I asked him what he wanted the money for.

"I can't tell you." he replied.

"Well honey," I said, "I can't take that kind of money out of the bank if I don't know what it's for."

"It's none of your business!" was his response. "It's my money!"

"Yes, I know it is," I said, "but I have to pay all the bills, and as it is, we're barely breaking even. You can buy whatever you want but I still need to know what it is you need, before I can get that kind of money."

Then he asked, "Well what about the servants? What do we pay them? How long is it since they've had a raise?"

"We don't need to worry on that score," I assured him, "as we don't have any servants. We couldn't afford them anyway!"

"So who does all the work around here then?" was his response.

"I do, of course," I replied.

"Well then," he continued, "How much do you get paid?"

"Nothing!" I replied. "I do it for love."

He scoffed at that, but ended the conversation by

suggesting that I should get a nice raise then. At least, by that time, he'd forgotten all about wanting the money.

Edwin sat down to put on his shoes one afternoon, removing his slippers to do so. He put on one shoe, and then began looking all over the house for the other one. It was still sitting beside his slippers where he'd put on the first shoe. I took him back to the chair and showed him the other shoe, which he then put on. However, once again I found him searching all over the house and asked what he was looking for this time.

"I can't find my slippers," was his reply.

Of course, they were still sitting right where he had taken them off.

That same evening he kept asking again, "Who runs this place?"

At least by then the slippers didn't matter anymore.

He was always packing his bag to leave for "home," wherever that might be. He would usually include his camera, along with whatever else he felt necessary to take with him that particular day. Once he packed two pairs of slippers, one pair of shoes, his pyjamas, and a cardigan vest before declaring he was ready to go. Another time it could be food, or chocolate bars, or even several shirts along with his camera. Each time was different, except that it almost always included his camera, his most prized possession. One day he asked me which bus he should take, or should he call a taxi? He was so insistent, I finally had to sit him down and try to explain things to him. Usually I would take him out for a walk, even if only around the block and back as I often did—or for a short drive in the car—but that day it was pouring rain and I really didn't want to go out in such inclement weather on a "fool's errand" to take him home, so I tried to reason with him.

"Just who do you think I am?" I asked him directly, slightly exasperated by then.

Poor Edwin looked stricken because he couldn't remember my name, but he finally replied, "The kindest, sweetest person I've ever known!"

How could I get upset with that answer? I couldn't think of anything else to say so I just hugged him, moved to tears by his response.

What more could I have said? It was so sweet—and yet, so sad. I just felt like crying all the time.

He just wanted to *go home*! A simple request on the surface, but where was home?

For him there was no tangible place left called "home." I suddenly realized the validity of that well-known saying, "Home is where your hat is." For Edwin, that had become almost a euphemism, for his home truly was *where his hat was*, wherever that might be. Home was where he happened to be living at any given time. He *was* home, but he just didn't know it!

Never again will I take home for granted. Home is our haven, a place where we can feel safe; where we're able to be ourselves, kick off our shoes, and relax. That is home, no matter how humble, and we all need such a place in our lives. Edwin needed his home—a place where he could feel safe and secure—but it was lost to him, forever!

His hat was still hanging in the closet by the front door, evidence that Edwin was *at home*—not unlike the flag that hangs above Buckingham Palace—if you will—indicating the Queen to be in residence; or the flags in the many embassies throughout the world that only fly when the house is occupied; or the flag flying above the White House in Washington, D.C. to indicate the presence of the President.

He was in residence; his house was occupied; he was *at home* because his hat was there—but he was not *home*. For him the flags had ceased to fly. His body was home, but Edwin didn't live there any more!

Respite!

CHAPTER 8

When I took my husband for one of his doctor's appointments, the doctor spoke to both of us again, of the need for Edwin to be in a nursing home where they could look after him twenty-four hours a day. Edwin wouldn't consider it, of course, and I agreed. The doctor continued to insist that I needed a rest and must get some help before I broke down myself. I realized the veracity of his sentiments, but had no idea where to turn for help, other than a nursing home, which was still out of the question as far as I was concerned.

During the course of that same visit, the doctor expressed a statement that helped to settle a lot of the confusion in my own mind about what I should be doing for Edwin and what was best for him.

He said, "Well, of course, Edwin has the right to refuse any treatment he wants. I'm only here, as a doctor, *not to keep him alive, but to keep him happy while he is alive.*"

I was surprised at his words, and the manner in which he envisioned his role in treating my husband. However, pondering it in my own mind, and considering the circumstances, I decided that I could live with such a goal as well. Thus I made up my mind, there and then, to dedicate my time to making Edwin as happy as possible for the time he had left. Realizing that nothing more could be done for him medically, there was no use prolonging the agony of subjecting him to any more tests and probing, which wouldn't help him anyway. There was no cure, so why not allow him to enjoy the time he had remaining in this life? Since there would be no more "quantity of life" for him, I promised myself that I would give him "quality of life" instead.

I also realized, however, that the doctor was right about my needing help. I knew I couldn't go on much longer the way I was, going without sufficient sleep, unable to eat properly, and constantly on edge. I was becoming a bundle of nerves and that wasn't going to help my husband at all. One of the doctors had suggested Respite Care and had given me the address to apply to Social Services and subsequently to their Alzheimer's Respite Service Department for consideration. After filling out the necessary papers of application and submitting them for their approval, arrangements were made to send someone out to assess our situation as soon as possible. There was no question of our qualifying for their services, and they promised to provide respite care for us, up to twelve hours a week.

Finally! It was a good start and I was very grateful. The cost was only $8.50 an hour at that time, the remainder being subsidized by the government, but it had to be done in increments of three hours, no less.

Edwin really balked at the suggestion of anyone but myself staying with him, even if only for three hours, while I went out. He couldn't understand, first of all, why I had to go anywhere without him. Then, secondly, why did he need a babysitter, since he'd been looking after himself for years? Anyway, why couldn't I have stayed with him? After all, I was his wife, and wives should always be with their husbands! That's the way it was! He didn't want anyone else! That's the way he saw the situation and he'd brook no argument to the contrary. Incidentally, in case you were wondering, that day he did know that I was his wife—obviously— although in that particular instance it might have been simpler if he hadn't known. I could never win with him! That's why it was so hard to believe it wasn't pre-meditated at times—yet I've been assured that it wasn't possible for him to plan or think things through in such a way. I'm sure I'll never really understand.

He made me feel so guilty even wanting a break, but I knew I had to fight against bearing that guilt as a burden. I couldn't let him lay that guilt on me, and I recognized that I could care for him better when I wasn't bound to him twenty-four hours a day, seven days a week! I only hoped that whoever they sent, it would be someone with whom Edwin could relate, someone he could talk to, and someone who would be understanding and patient with him.

Meanwhile, I was continuing to enjoy my early morning walks (especially since the weather was improving daily), using my monitors, and usually returning before Edwin would wake up. I still maintain that it was the daily walks that helped most to keep my sanity during all those trying months and years.

One evening, before we'd even considered the process of applying for Respite Care, and I had lived with Alzheimer's for over nine months without a break, my friend Pat took me to a concert with the Toronto Symphony Orchestra, while her husband Bill stayed with Edwin. That "double offering" was their birthday gift to me and I was thrilled. It was my first break in all that time and I was very grateful. The entire evening was wonderful and I thoroughly enjoyed every minute of it. On arriving home, I found that Edwin was still up, having refused to go to bed until I returned. When I asked him if he'd had a nice evening, he said "No," in a very surly tone. Actually, I suspect he really did enjoy his evening, as I knew Bill to be a great conversationalist, and I'd left them a lovely chili dinner, one of Edwin's favourite meals. However, I don't think he wanted to admit to having enjoyed it, much like a child would react, consciously or subconsciously perhaps, because it might encourage me to go away more often. Whatever his reasoning, I'm glad it went so well. It was a wonderful gift for me and I appreciated the willing sacrifice on Bill's part. To me, that was an act of true friendship, a giving of his time and effort, a gift worth far more than money could ever buy, and I was deeply grateful.

The following day Edwin absolutely drove me nuts, following me around the house like a puppy dog, while I was doing the laundry and other such chores. He didn't remember my having been away the previous evening, but obviously in the back of his mind he remembered the feelings of insecurity, evoked by my leaving him for that time. At any rate, he refused to let me out of his sight that day and I was constantly tripping over him, even more than usual.

At one point he was unable to grasp the fact that the laundry equipment belonged to us, as did the house. He kept thinking that we were only renting the place and all the equipment with it. It was rather strange really, as he still knew his home address perfectly, even the postal code (as well he should after more than 39 years), but he had no idea that the house we were in, actually was at that address. To him, the house we were living in at that time was still not his home. As I mentioned before, sometimes he'd think his home was in London, England and he would quote that address perfectly, but could not remember the Canadian one. However, that particular day it was the Canadian one he could recite, and not the one from his childhood in England.

That afternoon, while I was trying to make dinner and still tripping over Edwin at every turn, he asked about his doctor's appointment for the next day, wanting to know if it was in the same place or someplace closer.

Then he asked me, "Just how long have you been doing this?"

"Doing what?" I answered.

"Escorting people around," he said, "To doctors and things."

Something wasn't ringing true again so at that point I asked him, "Do you know who I am?"

He said, "Well I can't put an official name to what you are...."

"Fine," I said, "But then who am I—unofficially?"

He then replied, "Well, you're someone who helps people and takes them places." Then he thought for a minute and continued, "You care for people and know all the answers!"

I only wish I *had* known all the answers!

Later, during dinner that same evening, he asked me, "What sort of a reception did you get from the local *gendarmerie*?"

I said, "You mean the police?"

"Yes," he replied.

"Well, in what way do you mean?" I asked, grasping for some idea of his train of thought.

Then he explained.

"When you moved in here, did they ask you the usual questions? How long would you be staying?"

Trying to change the subject, I replied, "I'm staying as long as you need me."

However, still later he brought up the subject again, asking me, "Who runs this operation? Do the police run it?"

I'm not sure where he thought he was living, but at that stage he had no idea who I was and seemed to be under the illusion that he was in a detention centre or a facility of some sort, run by the police. Where such fancies stemmed from I had no idea.

At times like that I just felt scared and vulnerable myself. I never knew what he would do or say next. All I could do was try to keep him calm, and attempt to stay calm myself, which was almost as difficult. If possible, I tried never to argue with him and I'd go along with whatever conversation he initiated, steering it in safer directions if I could, although that wasn't always easy. In order to accomplish that, I would try to answer his questions, whenever feasible, in the way he wanted to hear them, and not in the way things really were. Of course in order to do that, I had to figure out his train of thought, which wasn't always possible. One thing was certain, there was no use in trying to correct him or point out the fallacy of his thinking. I could never have convinced him anyway, and trying to correct him or set him straight would often lead to aggression and anger on his part, a situation to be avoided at all cost. Believe me, I used to try, earlier on in his illness, but it only aggravated him and would open up a whole new line of questions, upsetting him unnecessarily, so I gave up trying. It was much better to go along with him whenever possible—better for both of us!

There were other questions he would ask, over and over again at times, but no answer was ever satisfactory to him.

"How did you get all our furniture here?" he would ask.

Also, "Why did you bring it here?"

Though he would revert to asking the same questions incessantly, and would return to previous topics on numerous occasions, every day it would be something different! Who said "variety is the spice of life?" At that point I'd have given anything for some plain, old, ordinary living—anything but the constant changes to our routine. In truth, nothing was routine any more, and life was just one hurdle after another, each one seeming higher and harder than the one before!

One evening Edwin declared that he wanted to go to the bank, and asked me for the bank statements. He wanted to withdraw a large sum of money but wouldn't tell me what it was for, except to say it was a surprise. Later on he told me that he had talked recently to a man who showed him how to invest money on the stock market so I asked him when he had spoken to this man.

"About ten days ago," was his reply.

I then asked where he had spoken to him.

He answered, "Downtown."

Of course he hadn't been downtown in over a year, and he certainly hadn't been anywhere without me, so I knew it was impossible. However, by then I was concerned that he might try to do something foolish. I didn't want to see him throwing away his money—not that he had a lot to throw away—but I also didn't want him to feel like his input didn't matter anymore, so I found a way to compromise. I took him to the bank and helped him withdraw a thousand dollars from the account, thankful that, to his way of thinking, this was a lot of money. Having regressed to the past as he had, a chocolate bar was only worth ten cents, in *his* mind at least, so this was indeed a huge sum! Actually, he was inordinately pleased with himself and his acquisition, and that seemed to satisfy him for the time. Later, when he had forgotten all about it, I removed the money from his wallet, before he could lose it or misplace it, and returned it to the bank. That method seemed to work very well, and continued to do so each time he would declare his need for a large sum of money, at which time we would repeat the same process all over again. That way he was quite happy and still felt in control of his own destiny and finances.

The day finally arrived when the representative for the Alzheimer's Respite Program came to our home to do the assessment. She was very nice and it went well, except for Edwin's insistence that he didn't want or need anyone to come in and he certainly didn't want me going out, but she understood where he was coming from, so didn't let it deter her. Before leaving she promised that help would be forthcoming, very soon. Edwin finally grasped the fact that someone else was going to come in to look after him from time to time, but in his mind he equated that with his perception of my intention to leave him permanently—or at least for a long time. I kept trying to reassure him that I had no intention of going away, other than for a few short hours, but it was difficult at best. He'd finally understand what I was saying, only to start the same thing all over again a short time later, having become convinced again that I was leaving him. And so it went....

One evening Edwin asked me to be frank with him and answer a question truthfully. Of course I agreed.

Then he asked, "How many people are looking after me?"

I answered, "Just myself...at least so far. Why do you ask?"

He went on to say, "I keep thinking there are three women here looking after me: one who looks after the flowers in the garden, one who does the cooking and one who looks after me and drives me places!"

In reply I said, "Well, I do the gardening and the cooking and I look after you. I'm your wife!"

Then he said, "But I keep thinking of my wife as somebody else."

Gently, I replied, "Maybe you're thinking of your first wife?"

"My first wife!" he exclaimed. "But you're my first wife, aren't you?"

"No, Trudy was your first wife," I explained.

"Trudy!" he reiterated, "Who's Trudy?"

I replied, "Trudy was your first wife. You seem to dwell in the past a lot, especially during your time in the war. Perhaps you're remembering Trudy from back then, when you were both young and very much in love, during your time in the Royal Air Force."

"Trudy," he said, thoughtfully, "I'd forgotten all about her."

He still had times of relative lucidity and we'd have

conversations like that during those occasions. He told me that he often thought I was someone else; the flower lady, as he'd put it, or the cook, or whatever else came to mind, but then he'd realize he was hallucinating. Then he confessed that most of the time his brain just seemed foggy and unclear. As much as they pained me, I also appreciated such conversations as they helped me to understand what he was going through himself.

A few days after that conversation, our first care-giver came in to stay with Edwin for three hours, while I went out to an Alzheimer's Support Group. (That was my very first time at such a meeting, though not my last, but I will deal with that subject later in this chapter.) Edwin was fine while I was gone, but I felt like I was going through withdrawal myself. The entire time I was away I kept worrying about him; wondering what he was doing, and hoping the care-giver could cope with him. I needn't have worried though, as he was fine. Of course he was very glad to see me when I arrived home, demonstrably so. Everything had been all right in my absence, the only incident being when Edwin told the care-giver he had to go to a meeting, and insisted she had to leave, after she'd only been there for a short while. Fortunately she was able to handle him. Apparently they talked about me a lot that evening but since Edwin couldn't remember my name, he'd just refer to me as his wife. At least he remembered that! I was encouraged.

Each time I would schedule a respite break, poor Edwin would almost spoil it for me by making me feel guilty for leaving him. He'd start in the morning, moping about the house and expressing his displeasure with me in eloquent body language, as well as verbally. The agency had suggested we work out a schedule so the care-giver could come on the same day and time each week. That way we could enjoy the continuity of having the same person coming, rather than subjecting Edwin to a different person each time. We settled on Thursday afternoons, as I had enrolled in an eight-week Care-giver's Seminar at the public library and it was held on Thursday afternoons. I looked forward to the break each week and tried not to let Edwin spoil it by laying a "guilt trip" on me, but it was never easy.

Another Thursday had rolled around and I was anticipating my afternoon off, but Edwin began first thing in the morning, as usual, asking me when I was coming back.

He would start by saying, "Now let me get this straight. You won't get back until midnight?"

The next time he'd say, "You aren't returning until 10 am tomorrow, right?"

Then five minutes later it would be, "So, you'll be away for 12 hours?"

On and on it went! I got so frustrated answering him every five minutes that I finally wrote him a note saying I would be away for *only* three hours. Then, whenever he'd ask me again, I'd say, "Read the note!"

That helped a lot, except that he kept losing the note, as he'd put it away in a different pocket each time he read it. Sometimes I'd just want to scream when he'd carry on like that. He would pout and sulk all day, whenever I went away, declaring that I couldn't love him or I wouldn't leave him like that. I'd usually end up feeling so sick and miserable, I'd wonder if the break was worth it, going through that hassle every time.

After my care-giver's course was finished I found myself at loose ends on those Thursday afternoons. Sometimes I'd go to a movie with Alma when she was available, but mostly I'd just wander around the mall. I couldn't go home for three hours and even though it doesn't seem like a long time, it can feel interminable when you have nothing to do. I knew I needed the break and I did appreciate being able to get out on my own, but I'd wander around the mall, since the weather wasn't conducive to being outside, worrying about my husband, wondering if he was missing me, and feeling guilty for having left him. I couldn't afford to shop, except for a few necessities, and I'd hope by some off-chance to run into someone I knew so I could justify stopping for a coffee.

I should interject here to say how warped one's thinking can become when one is subjected to such situations, day in and day out. I deserved a break! If I wanted to stop for a leisurely coffee, I deserved that luxury! That was my time, time to myself, time to breath, time to enjoy, but somehow—somewhere along the way—I had lost the ability to enjoy myself.

This is a natural phenomenon, in cases such as mine, and I'm sure many people will be able to identify with me in feeling the same way. However, it is something to be avoided nonetheless. We, as care-givers, can become so wrapped up in our world of caring for our loved one, who is suffering, that in trying to take the burden from them, we put it on ourselves. Until we realize this, we can never be free of the burden of guilt, which can be devastating, believe me! Therefore, unless we're willing to face this issue, and consciously accept what we are doing, there will never be any help for us. I can't emphasize this problem enough and I must warn you not to allow yourself to fall into such a deadly trap.

One Thursday, after the care-giver had been with Edwin all afternoon, my husband kept referring to the care-giver as "they" when I asked him about his afternoon's activities. I tried to explain to him that there had only been one person there with him, but he was convinced there had been at least two. He told me that "they" kept asking him questions about how he came to own his house. Trying to humour him, and change the subject, I asked what he had told them in answer to their questions.

"Oh I told them lots of stories!" he replied.

"What kind of stories?" I asked.

"Oh I don't know," he said, "I just made them up as I went along!"

"Why would you do that?" I wanted to know.

"Because I didn't know what they wanted me to say," was his reply.

After that he commented on the fact that he couldn't get over 'our having the same pictures and furniture.' I asked him what he was talking about and he explained that he had gone to another house, completely foreign to him, but they had exactly the same pictures and furniture as our house. Obviously this occurred in his mind, when he and the care-giver returned home from their walk, and his house had appeared strange to him, as though he'd arrived at another house, instead of returning to the same one.

Some time later, while attending the Alzheimer's Seminar for Care-givers, I learned about Day Programs for people like Edwin, enabling the patient to spend the entire day with others like themselves, participating in organized activities and giving the care-givers a break from 9:00 a.m. to 4:00 p.m. As well, of course, the activities helped to use up a lot of the patients' seemingly boundless energies, ultimately making them easier to handle in the evening. (Nowadays, even night programs are available in some cities for those patients who don't sleep at night, giving their care-givers a chance to get some much-needed rest.) With the help of the seminar leader, I applied for Edwin to enter such a Day Program. Again, a representative was sent over to our home in order to assess Edwin and our situation, before he was admitted to the group. That having been accomplished, he was assigned two days a week that he could attend the Day Program, and it made a welcome change for me. It gave me a chance to do some necessary chores that were being neglected while I was so tied up with my husband all day. As well, it made the housework so much easier to accomplish without having him underfoot. It also enabled me to catch up on some needed rest and relaxation, something that had become rather scarce since our initial introduction to Alzheimer's.

The first day there, I attended the Alzheimer's Day School with Edwin, remaining with him the entire day and taking part in all the activities, and I was very impressed with the program. The facilities were also great, as was the quality of care and the school personnel were wonderful. One thing I did notice, that first day at the program, involved Edwin's participation (or lack thereof) in some of the programs and games. For the most part, he had neither a clue as to what was going on, nor the knowledge of what was expected of him in order to participate. It appeared that the other patients had much better mental abilities and acuity than did Edwin, and I was concerned at how far he'd deteriorated in so short a time. However, that aspect of things entirely aside, Edwin fit in beautifully with the other patients and I was certain, given time, he'd adjust very well. *Time* was the operative word, of course, as I knew it would take some time for him to get used to the idea of not having me around all day, every day.

Unfortunately, by five o'clock when we arrived home that first day, he had become confused and disorientated again, convinced that someone else had driven him home—and stolen all his things. Nothing was missing, of course, but he wouldn't accept that as proof. At such times, it was becoming increasingly difficult to handle him. However, I knew the day had been trying for him—not that he didn't enjoy it, but it had all been so new and different—so I tried to be as patient with him as possible, understanding how confused he must feel. I know it was difficult enough for me, but I just can't imagine how awful it must have been for him!

On returning to the Day School the next time, Edwin walked right in with no problem, but became very upset when I left, refusing to eat. However, the care-givers told me afterwards that he became quite sociable as the day wore on. When I arrived to pick him up that afternoon, he was so glad to see me, he walked towards me, with tears in his eyes, and his arms outstretched, like a young child to his mother. It was rather touching and I couldn't control a tear or two of my own as I hugged him tenderly. In fact, I noticed several of the workers wiping their eyes as well.

The remainder of that evening he continued to rave about how wonderful I was, and how lucky he was to have me, and how I took such good care of him.

He kept saying, "I never realized how lucky I was until I almost lost you!" (Nothing like a little deprivation to make you appreciate what you have! This insight, perhaps, just might be something to keep in mind!)

The sentiments were sweet and I did treasure them. It was nice to be appreciated for a change, if only briefly. However, after a while it became suffocating, as he wouldn't let me out of his sight, even for a moment.

Once Edwin was well established in the Day Program, attending regularly two days a week, the doctor decided it was time to try him on a new medication to see if it would improve his behaviour. He didn't expect any obvious changes to be evident for at least a week, but I began to see real improvement in only two days. I know for myself I wanted to be convinced that he was getting better, so I probably wasn't completely impartial in my judgment; however, when others also noticed positive improvement, I felt justified in my observations, and overjoyed. That Friday, even the staff at the Alzheimer's Day Program commented on Edwin being totally changed, a completely different person from the agitated individual he had usually been. They were really pleased with him and impressed with the results of the new medication. It seemed to be doing wonders for him and I was thrilled.

At this point you may be wondering why I'm not revealing the name of the new drug and pushing its use. The reason I'm not doing that is twofold. I am not writing this book to promote any form of treatment or medication, nor do I profess to be an expert in dealing with this disease in any way. I am only an ordinary person, thrust into an extraordinary situation, not of my choosing and certainly not in my line of expertise. What I have learned, I have gained through my experiences, my failures, and my successes. This book is strictly a non-medical, personal account of my experiences in dealing with one person, my husband, in his journey through this devastating disease. If by writing it I can help even one person traveling the same road, then it will have been worth all the time and effort I've contributed to this account.

As mentioned in the preceding paragraph, my reasons were twofold. The second reason I am not revealing the name of the drug is that, although it made such a radical change in my husband, it's benefits were short-lived at best. As his agitation settled down, and the fog in his mind began to clear somewhat, eventually his entire personality changed. While he had been agitated before, he now became aggressive and angry, and as the fog cleared, he began to hallucinate more, in radically different ways. Thus we realized, to our disappointment and dismay, as far as the Alzheimer's disease was concerned, there were still no miracles—at least not yet! Hopefully this will change in the future, but for us it was not to be.

Some mornings Edwin would go to his Day Program in a very bad mood, which wouldn't improve during the course of the day. Unfortunately, his temper did nothing to ameliorate the situation either, and as the day wore on, he would make a real nuisance of himself, throwing tantrums and creating scenes. I marveled at the ability of the care-givers to cope with him, along with everyone else, on days like that especially, and admired the patience those wonderful workers displayed in caring for such difficult people, day after day. I felt an overwhelming gratitude to them, and others like them, for their willingness to share their time and their talents, indeed, their very lives, in such a thankless profession. Truly these are some of God's "Angels" on earth.

One such day, when poor Edwin was unhappy with the world at large, he was still crabby and irritable when I picked him up after school. I realized he must have had a bad day too, as his clothing was also in disarray when I arrived, and he'd brook no assistance in rearranging it, neither from me, nor anyone else. All the way home he complained about *slave labour*! It seems that it was his turn to help with the lunch dishes that day!

Other times he'd refer to the Day School as "going to work." Actually, that wasn't so bad, as he enjoyed going to work because it made him feel needed and important. The only thing he objected to was the fact that he *never got paid*! He just couldn't understand why. Apparently the staff at the school would ask him questions about his service in the Royal Air Force, and he loved relating stories to them of his experiences in India during the war, and Germany after the war, where he did aerial reconnaissance and aerial photography for the R.A.F. However, he'd maintain that the people at the Day Centre were "deprogramming" him by asking him to relate all these tales, and that he was working as a spy for his country. Thus his "job" involved answering all their questions and giving them "inside information" on the war effort.

It worked for me! Whatever kept him happy was fine with me. Even so, though he enjoyed going to work, there were many days as well, when he was not so eager to attend, and would refuse to get into the car at all. Finally, I stopped telling him where we were going and I'd just take him for a ride in the car. When we'd end up at the school he'd usually walk in quite happily, having no idea where he was, as the building was new to him each time we arrived. That is certainly one advantage with Alzheimer's, as their inability to recognize people and places makes it much easier to get them to certain locations when they don't wish to go there.

Now a chapter on Respite Care would not be complete if I did not deal with one other aspect of Respite, that of Alzheimer's Support Groups. These groups fulfill a real need among care-givers and family members of those suffering from dementia, and everyone can benefit from what they have to offer. I certainly enjoyed many benefits from attending my support group, and will always be grateful for their help. In fact, through the years of caring for Edwin, I attended regularly, once a month, often finding help and encouragement from the group, although just as often being able to help others by sharing my own experiences with them. Each of us had opportunity to help others in the group, if only by way of encouragement, but usually we'd find ourselves equally encouraged as well, by those among the gathering.

Initially, for me at least, the single most beneficial element I gleaned from attending a support group was to learn that *I was not alone!* I was not alone in traveling that long, dark road I had embarked on when my husband contracted this terrible disease. Hundreds of thousands had travelled that road ahead of me, and thousands more would follow, but none of us was alone! What a comfort it was to realize that I was not the only one going through that nightmare. Not that I would have wished the experience on anyone else of course, but just knowing that others had been there before me, helped to lift that terrible load from my shoulders, and what a relief it was. Nothing had changed really, but everything had changed for me. I was not alone!

I was not alone!

Somehow, that made all the difference in the world to me. I received many other benefits from attending the support group as well, finding help and encouragement for my desperate need, learning of new methods and of new drugs to help combat the disease, and finding the strength I needed to carry on. We enjoyed videos, which taught us a lot about Alzheimer's and what to expect in the future; special speakers who visited us from various organizations dealing with dementia; and even doctors, specialists, who shared with us their expertise on the subject.

Of course, no one has all the answers, but everyone had good ideas to share at our meetings as well. What worked for one person might not work for another, but the sharing of successful methods used by some, and the not-so-successful attempts by others, all contributed to that feeling of camaraderie as we gleaned some greater understanding of the disease, and how to deal with it in our everyday lives.

Karen, for instance, who lovingly tended to the needs of her father-in-law during his years with Alzheimer's, related the story of his love for one particular sweater. It was a yellow sweater and he never wanted to wear anything else. Rather than facing a fight over his daily apparel, she and Al solved the problem by going out and buying several yellow sweaters, all the same, so that Al's father could wear what he wanted but still have a clean sweater each day. A simple solution, yes, but it served to avoid a daily conflict. In fact, since Edwin also enjoyed wearing certain clothing more than others, I tried adopting a similar method for him, with great success. It also helped when he'd soil his clothing, as I'd only have to remove the part that needed laundering, rather than having to change him completely in order to coordinate his outfit. By creating a mix-and-match wardrobe for him I ended up saving myself a lot of extra work and hassle. Thus we learned, one from the other, different ways of dealing with the inherent problems of the disease, and more effective methods of coping with the stress.

Through those long years I also recommended the meetings to others just starting the journey with Alzheimer's. So often they would claim, as did I, that they were not ready yet for such a group. However, I would urge them, always, not to wait until they felt ready. In fact, I don't think anyone is ever ready! The time to go to such a group is before you think you need it. When you need it, it's already too late. I've found in life that it is so much easier to face things when you know what you're facing. Knowing is half the battle. I've always felt that I could face anything life had to offer, if I only knew what it was. It's the not knowing that can be so frightening! I would never want anyone to go through what I did, feeling so alone out there in Florida, and not knowing what was happening to us. Knowledge is power, and learning can instill that power in your heart and in your hands, enabling you to face the future, and to face each day as it comes.

There are many support groups out there and I urge all care-givers to seek one out in your area. If you don't like the one you find, then try another. If there isn't one in your area then why not start your own? It might surprise you how well-received it could be.

Even now, as I meet people from day to day, I wonder how many of them are hurting, facing difficult, even unbearable, challenges as they go through life, hiding their pain behind a smile—or a scowl—and perhaps already nearing the end of their rope. There is a great need out there, and if we can help to alleviate even some small part of it, our being here has not been in vain. Even our own painful experiences and suffering will not have been for naught, if they can be used to help another along that same pathway. I know I shall never again take happiness for granted! It comes with a price!

I shall always be grateful for the support group I found, and for the help and encouragement it gave to me during those long, dark days of living with Alzheimer's. I am also grateful for those who gave of themselves to lead the group, sacrificing their time and energy to help those in need. They will always have a very special place in my heart.

Sound the Alarm!

CHAPTER 9

At times Edwin would forget where he was and become convinced he should be somewhere else. That could be anywhere, such as going home, going to the store or to the bank, or going to work. However, most of the time, I could usually waylay him by encouraging him in another direction, or if all else failed, by going with him. Then we'd simply go for a walk around the block, or for a short drive in the car, if the weather was not conducive to walking, and by the time we'd return home, in most cases, he'd have forgotten his mission, or he'd think we had arrived at his goal. Of course, if his original quest had been to go home, which was most often the case, I'd just announce that we were home again, and wasn't it good to be there, or something equally inane, and it usually worked.

However, what concerned me were the times he would try to leave by himself, to pursue his mission alone, and those times had started to become more frequent. I did have to attend to my own personal needs on occasion and he seemed to know just when I'd be otherwise occupied. I could step into the bathroom for two minutes and find him missing when I came out, or I could be involved with making dinner and not watching him as carefully as usual. Also, some nights I would become so exhausted from lack of sleep that I wouldn't always hear him when he got out of bed. At any rate, I realized I had to do something about it before he got hurt or lost. I bought him an ID bracelet and registered him with the Alzheimer's Wandering Registry, which was a good start. They are an excellent organization, providing a necessary service, and I do recommend them highly, but I still needed to do more in order to set my mind at ease. My greatest fear was that my husband might injure himself before he was found and I could not take that chance. I investigated all my options and at length decided to invest in an alarm system that would ring, when set, whenever the front door was opened. It also provided a motion sensor, which could be set separately, so I could know if he ventured anywhere near the basement stairs, which were of great concern to me as well. This actually proved very effective for us, as long as I remembered to set the alarm; which I didn't always do during the day, as I needed to be able to go in and out myself on occasion. However, I always set it at night and it worked most efficiently.

One night after Edwin had gone to sleep, I fell into a particularly deep sleep, totally exhausted from a trying day and several frustrating nights of very little sleep. Usually a light sleeper, that night I was out for the count and not aware of Edwin slipping out of bed. Suddenly I was rudely awakened by an awful, shrieking siren! I jumped out of bed and raced into the living room to find poor Edwin standing in the middle of the room, shaking with fear.

"What happened?" I asked, after turning off the alarm.

"I went to the bathroom and lost myself!" was his pathetic reply.

He looked so forlorn and was cowering like a lost child, so I just hugged him for a long time, before taking him off to bed again. Poor soul, I guess the alarm really frightened him.

I know it scared me!

During the day I usually left the alarm turned off, as I was often in and out the door myself, either going into the garden or out back to cook something on the barbecue. In most cases I would take Edwin with me, but at times I would just pop out to take the garbage, or sweep the walk, or even shovel the snow in winter, so I could not take him along. On those occasions Edwin's paranoia would often take over and he'd lock the door behind me. This happened so many times that I had to make a point of always carrying a key in my pocket. However, sometimes locking the door wasn't enough to satisfy him, and he'd lock the screen door as well. The only problem there was that the screen door didn't have a key! It could only be unlocked from the inside! I'd then have to knock and knock on the door before he'd let me in. One day though, knocking on the door didn't suffice to rouse him and he didn't come to open it for me. I'd been shovelling the driveway and was wet and cold, so after knocking for a while, I finally resorted to banging and pounding on the door, but still to no avail. I couldn't seem to get him to respond at all. In the end I had to go over to the neighbour's house and telephone home, asking him please to open the door so I could get in. After that episode I actually broke the lock on the screen door deliberately, so he couldn't lock me out again. I wasn't taking any more chances!

One day I was out in the back yard painting the fence. Edwin asked if he could do anything to help so I handed him a set of two keys and some money I had in my pocket, asking him to put them on the kitchen counter for me. Instead of doing as I'd asked, he put both items in his wallet. Then, not five minutes later, he pulled the keys out of his wallet again, claiming he had just discovered them and wondering where they had come from. My money was also in his wallet but he had absolutely no recollection of my having given either the money or the keys to him. He just thought he'd made a great find!

My brother and his wife were coming from Arizona for a visit shortly after that, and I had agreed to meet them for lunch at a nearby restaurant. I figured it would be much easier to visit there without the distractions of home. Edwin absolutely refused to go with me, so I arranged a sitter for him. However, after lunch I brought my brother and his wife back to the house for coffee and a visit with Edwin. He was in a surly mood when we arrived and my brother's visit did nothing to improve it. In fact, he was very rude to them, and later started swearing and cursing, saying he wanted them out of his house immediately. They had done nothing wrong and were rather shocked at his behaviour. I was just very embarrassed for them all. Fortunately my brother was very understanding, realizing my husband's condition, and forgave us readily. I didn't understand it at all though, and was very upset. He'd never treated anyone that badly before, and anyway, why did it have to be my own brother? However, when I tried to speak to Edwin about his behaviour he was unrepentant. In fact, he was downright belligerent, expressing his dislike of my brother in no uncertain terms.

He finished his tirade by stating, "Well if this is what your relatives are like, I won't be married to you for long!"

I couldn't understand why he took such an instant dislike to my brother, unless his size intimidated him somehow. (My brother is 6'2"). At any rate, even though I knew in my heart that Edwin was not responsible for his actions, in that particular case I felt very bad, and totally humiliated. This was my family, my flesh and blood, whom I hadn't seen for several years, and this is how they were treated in my home. The entire performance was extremely degrading and left me feeling very bitter. I really had a hard time forgiving Edwin for what he'd done, even though I knew it wasn't his fault, and I realized how imperfect and very human I was. However, when I shared the story with my friend Alma, she helped me to see the situation in an entirely different light. She suggested that perhaps Edwin was just jealous of my brother, since he'd known me a lot longer than Edwin had. Of course, why hadn't I thought of that? Edwin was jealous of anyone or anything that took my attentions away from him, so he was bound to be jealous of my brother, who already had a prior claim on my life. Understanding that made it much easier for me to forgive the offence.

Later that year my daughter Melissa and her husband David came to Toronto for a few days holiday and reunion with all of David's relatives, so I arranged for a sitter and planned to meet them at their hotel for a nice visit. I certainly wasn't going to make the same mistake of bringing them home to visit Edwin, knowing what to expect in that direction. The hotel where they were staying was very elegant and beautifully appointed, conveniently situated in downtown Toronto within walking distance from all the major attractions. However, I was especially impressed by the fact that each of the guest rooms had a telephone located in the bathroom—would you believe it—of all places! Since I'd promised to call Edwin from the hotel on my arrival, I just couldn't resist using that particular phone.

When he came on the line I said to him, "You'll never guess where I'm phoning from...the bathroom!"

I could hear Edwin's voice brighten perceptibly as he replied.

"Our bathroom!!"

After that everyone wondered why I was laughing so hard...in the bathroom!

One evening Edwin was in a very surly mood, asking the same questions over and over, and complaining about everything and sundry. I was so glad when it finally came time to go to bed, as I'd had enough! However, that night he sat on the edge of the bed for a long time, looking sad and dejected, so I sat down beside him and put my arm around his shoulders.

"What's wrong, love? Why are you looking so sad?" I asked gently.

"What I want to know is," he said, forlornly, pausing momentarily, "where is my wife?"

Of course I hastened to assure him I was right there beside him. I just found it so sad that he didn't know who I was most of the time by then. However, the important thing was that he knew I was there to look after him (whoever I was), and he knew that I cared about him, and if that's all I could be to him any more, then so be it. I just knew I could never desert him.

One morning he tried to put on his cardigan vest by putting his head through the armhole. He realized he'd done something wrong but couldn't figure out what was amiss. Of course, as usual, it was always the fault of the clothing, not him! Every day something would be inside out or backwards. Once he even buttoned up his vest inside out so the strip with the buttons on it was sticking straight out front.

When I pointed this out to him his only comment was to say, "I thought it buttoned up strangely."

His ability to dress himself was gradually deteriorating and I realized that eventually I would have to do it all for him. However, I still persisted in my efforts to let him do things for himself as long as humanly possible. Whatever happened to my "snappy dresser" who was always impeccably turned out? How he would decry the caricature of himself he had become. It was a good thing he didn't know what had happened to him—what was happening still!

As an erstwhile professional photographer, Edwin had become used to wearing a cord on his glasses, to enable him to drop them at a moment's notice in order to look through the viewfinder of his camera. Thus, over the years, the cord had become a basic feature of his dress. I seldom saw him without the cord around his neck but it was muted and tasteful and never blatantly obvious. In fact, he'd always been a very smart dresser, impeccably elegant and well groomed, even in casual clothes, opting usually for tweed jackets with a shirt or turtleneck. That was also one of the things I'd always admired about him, his timeless taste in clothing and the ability to wear them with style.

However, one day when I handed him the cord for his glasses, he asked me what it was for, what he was supposed to do with it. I was stunned! I attempted to explain but he still didn't understand so I put it on his glasses for him. More and more he was losing his recognition of simple, everyday items he had always used, such as the cord for his glasses, and I noted each incidence with dread, as it marked yet another step down on his inexorable descent into the unknown. On another occasion I discovered him trying to tie that same cord to his slippers, for whatever reason I couldn't ascertain.

Whenever we went to the grocery store I would let Edwin help packing the bags, (except for the eggs of course), and he seemed to enjoy doing it. One day, however, I'd bought more than usual and he was having difficulty fitting them all in. Obviously trying to be helpful, he decided to get rid of the excess and threw them into the trash bin. Fortunately I saw him do it so I quickly ran over to rescue our purchases from the garbage. The clerk, who had served us, watched the entire scenario and laughed heartily, thinking it was hilarious, as I scrambled madly in their garbage can, trying to retrieve our groceries. Edwin had no idea what he found so funny, but laughed along with him. I didn't think it was at all funny, so I didn't laugh—at least not then!

Another grocery store fiasco involved the time Edwin took all the groceries that the cashier had already checked through the till, and put them back into the grocery basket, forcing us to redo the entire process again. The clerk wasn't very pleased with us, but I refused to pay twice for the same groceries so he had no choice. Poor Edwin thought he was helping! He just couldn't understand why we couldn't take the basket home with us too. He thought we'd bought it as well!

One night Edwin was searching high and low for his watch, which he wore every day, and I told him it was on his arm, as usual.

"No, not that one." he responded. "I'm looking for the long, thin one!"

It turned out he was looking for his pen but couldn't remember the correct word. Another time he was very proud of me because I had grouted the bathroom floor all by myself. However, he told everyone that I had fixed the ceiling. More often than not by that time, he would use the opposite word to the one he wanted, so I'd have to try and guess about what he actually was referring to, in most cases. It wasn't always easy!

Speaking of floors, on a particularly nice day I decided to wash the kitchen floor, which job was long overdue, I might add. After applying the wax, I asked Edwin not to walk on it until it was dry. However, even that simple request was too much for him to grasp, although he did remember my admonition. Somehow he decided that he couldn't walk anywhere in the rest of the house, except for the kitchen! Then he kept walking, through the kitchen, to find me and confirm that he'd understood it correctly.

"I shouldn't walk in the living room, right? But the kitchen is okay?"

Of course the floor was ruined by then but I gave up trying to explain it to him. I decided my sanity was worth more than the floors!

A Horse of a Different Colour

CHAPTER 10

The nightmare I was living in those days just continued to get worse and at times I'd find myself at my wits' end. In fact, I was beginning to fear that I'd break down myself, if I didn't learn how to handle the stress. The burden was almost intolerable! It felt as though a lump was growing in my chest, restricting my breathing and making it impossible to eat much of anything. Even my throat felt constricted and when I swallowed it felt like bile, rising from my stomach and burning my throat. When I did fall asleep in exhaustion, it was only to wake a short time later, painfully aware of the burden on my chest and in my heart, weighing me down, dragging me further and further into the pit of despair. At times I felt like giving up, but I knew I couldn't. Some days I just wanted to die, but I couldn't do that either because I knew my husband needed me. Even though he no longer knew who I was, he still needed me, and that thought—that knowledge alone—kept me going. Some days I thought I was dead...but then the pain would come again and I'd know I was still alive—not living—but alive!

By that time it seemed that Edwin was hallucinating more and more as well. One day, convinced there was a bunch of people on our patio at the side of the house, he wanted me to shoo them away. He went on and on about it so I finally told him to go and tell them himself to go away.

"They won't listen to me!" he'd complain, "but they will listen to you!"

I'm glad *he* was confident of my ability. I sure wasn't, but it was nice to know that someone thought me to be strong. Believe me I didn't feel strong at all any more. Quite the reverse!

Then another day, he kept seeing his late wife (who had died a number of years before), all over the house. This had never happened before. In fact, he'd never even talked about her previously, at least not since he'd acquired the Alzheimer's disease. However, that day his son had phoned to say that it would have been their anniversary, if his mom had still been alive! That was all it took to get him started! I just wish his son hadn't said anything, as after that comment, I had to live with the consequences. It would only take one word, one picture, one item, or even something on the TV to get him started down a certain road. From then on his grasp of the subject would be tenacious and he'd hang on to it "ad nauseum." Usually this happened in regard to wanting something he couldn't have, or looking for something he couldn't find, but in this case it was seeing someone from the past. Most of the time, of course, I wanted him to remember things, but those times I'd wish he would forget, but he never did. He'd just go on and on (like the proverbial Energizer Bunny) until his batteries would run down—or my patience. On those occasions, however, his endurance would be phenomenal and I would run down long before he did. By then I'd be a bundle of nerves myself.

That particular day I finally said to him, "I wish you'd show me where she is the next time you see her, because I have a few questions I'd like to ask of her."

Edwin replied, "I have a few questions for her too!"

However, following that conversation she refused to appear again!

There were many days when Edwin would not speak at all. Those times he would just sit there, blankly staring into space and seeing nothing at all. Whereas he used to doze a lot throughout the day, during our time in Florida at least, he seemed to have passed on to another stage at this point, where he seldom dozed at all. When he would decide to talk, he'd go on non-stop, giving long dissertations but usually saying nothing of any import— nothing that made any sense at any rate. It was often a mixture of many subjects, past and present, all rolled into one speech. For example, one such discourse went as follows:

"Everything is so complicated nowadays. Even going to bed. When I was this age, many years ago, all I needed was a match box with matches in it."

I had no idea what prompted that particular comment, much less what it meant, but it was a typical example of something he would say, a narration that would most often pop out of the blue with him, coming from nowhere, and leading to no obvious conclusion as well.

Another time, just as we were going to bed, Edwin made a comment about dogs, of all things, not that we had any!

He said, "I certainly hope you're not planning on calling out names as you start rounding up all those dogs!"

"What dogs?" I asked.

"All those bloody dogs you're going to be rounding up!" was his indignant reply.

Obviously he thought I should know what he was talking about but I hadn't a clue. Most of his stories or comments came out of left field, at least from my perspective, so I never knew how to respond exactly. If I made the correct retort, I could often keep the conversation going for quite a while, but the wrong response would only upset him or shut him up entirely, almost like talking to someone in his sleep!

Some days were harder than others, but they were all difficult, and many times I'd be on the verge of tears all day, crying myself to sleep that night. Each new dawn brought it's own set of horrors or nightmares, and just when I'd think it couldn't get any worse, it would! I was tired, worn out, and frustrated; too tired to sleep, even if Edwin didn't keep me awake half the night, and too much on edge to be able to relax any more. As it was, when this nightmare was finally over for me, I actually had to learn how to sleep all over again, having lost the ability to do so, during those long, dark years. In fact, to this day, sleeping is still difficult for me.

I was constantly amazed by Edwin's ability to tell stories, not true ones mind you, but plausible nonetheless. He'd take a wild mix of facts and fantasy, weave them all together, and build a believable, though somewhat incredulous story. Even though they were only make-believe stories, I could hardly correct him in the middle of his telling them, so I'd just have to let it go. As it was, I could never be sure whether people actually believed him or not, or if they recognized it as the ramblings of a confused, if credible, storyteller. Perhaps he even believed the stories himself? Who knows?

One day he started off talking about the x-ray he'd had of his neck. (He did have an x-ray to check his carotid artery at one stage, looking for any signs of a stroke, of which, thankfully, there were none.) He then finished up talking about stuffing dog biscuits into a sack. Don't ask me how he got there! I haven't a clue, but it all sounded rather convincing, even if it didn't make any sense.

Another time he told the story of how he was staying at a nursing home—or boarding school, I'm not sure which—where they were made to strip off all their clothes and stand naked while the staff flogged them. I certainly hope no one believed that I would actually do something like that to him! In fact, I doubt if anyone ever did that to him in his entire life—and I know they certainly never did any such thing in the nursing home where he finally lived—but there you have it! He seemed to believe it anyway.

Other times he would be convinced that someone was going to break into our home. On one such occasion he questioned me about it.

"Are there any busters that might try to charge in?" he asked.

"What are you talking about?" I replied, rather perplexed.

He became visibly upset and said, rather forcefully, "With tickets to the Woolworth Company, of course!"

One minute he could sound almost normal, but the next he'd be talking nonsense. The trouble was, I couldn't understand what he was trying to say or convey to me and that would upset him even more. It must have been terribly frustrating for him as well, trying to express his sentiments, but not succeeding. That type of conversation often seemed to occur, at least at the beginning of the disease, following a nap—whether a long one or just a quick shut-eye—so at times I'm sure it must have related to some extension of a dream, although he always claimed that he never dreamed, even when he was normal.

Expanding on that theory, I have noticed a distinct similarity during some of his strange conversations, between those interactions with Edwin and conversing with someone who is talking in their sleep. I do not know if there is a real parallel there or if I am making it up out of whole cloth but I definitely did detect a similarity between the two, enough to convince me there could be a connection, at least metaphorically. If there is a case for juxtaposition it could explain a lot of things. The questions remain then, yet to be answered: Are they actually living in a dream world or is this their reality? Is it really a nightmare—or "a horse of a different colour?" Perhaps we'll never know for sure.

I recall an incident that happened many years ago, when I was pregnant with my second daughter, Cynthia. I suffered from the usual anxieties associated with pregnancy, one of them for me being the fear of going to the bathroom alone in the middle of the night. To give you a better perspective, let me explain that we were living in the basement of an old country church and our bathroom was also the public washroom, located at the bottom of the stairs leading up to the church proper. The stairwell was long and unlit, the church building creaky and dark, and the whole scenario seemed rather menacing to me at that time, especially in the middle of the night! At any rate, in order to face this ordeal every night, I would have to awaken my poor husband to escort me. One day, my husband had worked long and hard on a frustrating electrical problem, which he was finally able to solve after several hours. It should have been an easy task, but it turned out to be long and frustrating, solved by the simple installation of a ground wire.

If he said it once that evening, he said it a dozen times, "All it needed was a ground wire! That's all it needed—just a ground wire!"

That night I woke him up as usual saying, "Honey, wake up. I need to go to the bathroom."

"But you can't go," he replied, still half asleep.

"Why can't I go?" I asked.

He answered, "You can't go to the bathroom, because you need a ground wire on the toilet!"

Looking back on that story still makes me smile. However, I can't help making an analogy between that incident and some of the conversations I'd had with Edwin during his years with Alzheimer's disease. Is there a connection? I don't know, but I do know that at times, talking with Edwin was almost like talking with someone still immersed in a dream. When a person dreams, it's usually based on the underlying frustrations or focal point of the preceding day, mixed in with all the multitude of other ingredients from that day, until it becomes one story, meshed together to form one continuous dream. Isn't that essentially what occurs with Alzheimer's patients? All the things they see and hear get jumbled up together in their minds, both past and present, side by side with fantasy and future, until they convince themselves and the dream becomes reality—for them at least!

There is one basic difference though, and I feel constrained to point it out. After my husband had that dream, all those years ago, *he woke up!*

One Day at a Time

"Where should I sleep tonight?" The same question recurred nightly by then, even though we had only one bedroom with a bed in it. The other two bedrooms had been converted into dens long ago, one for me and my music equipment and sewing machine, and the other with the television, where we sat together most evenings. For over 39 years my husband had slept in the same bedroom, on the same side of the bed and now he had to ask, not only where he should sleep but on which side of the bed as well. It was so hard to accept the fact that he really didn't know, even from one day to the next.

As usual, by that time, I would lead him to the bedroom and show him our bed, indicating which side was his. Then I would leave him to crawl under the covers while I went into the bathroom to take care of my own ablutions. One night, however, after I had left him to get into bed, my husband suddenly appeared in the doorway of the washroom, clearly agitated.

I asked him what was wrong and he replied, "You know that bed you told me about? Well, I can't sleep there."

"Why not?" I asked, puzzled, since this was the first time he'd refused.

Then he explained. "I can't sleep in there because there are already two ladies in the bed."

"Well," I replied, sounding more confident than I felt, I'm sure, "We'll just have to do something about that!"

Not bothering to argue with him, which would have been nothing more than an exercise in futility, I marched into the bed room and, raising my voice to an authoritative level, spoke to those (imaginary) ladies.

"Okay, ladies," I said, "it's time to leave! Off you go! My husband has to sleep now and he needs the bed so you'll just have to leave!"

Then I turned to Edwin and said, "Okay, they're gone now. You can go to bed."

And he did!

The next morning I figured he'd have forgotten all about it, but he hadn't! Once in awhile he'd surprise me by remembering something that happened the day before, and this was one of those times.

"You know those ladies that were in the bed last night?" he said, in quite a matter-of-fact tone. "Well, they left their teeth behind. There's a pair here for you too!"

So saying he handed me his false teeth. I took them, of course, (no sense arguing) and thanked him.

Actually it gave me an opportunity to clean them before returning them to him. (I tried to take advantage of every opportunity offered—in any category.) Later I returned his clean teeth to him and he popped them into his mouth without comment. As I said before, some of the anecdotes on his behaviour were quite funny—laughable even—if I'd felt like laughing!

On another occasion he was quite upset because there was a "bunch of people" in the living room, playing cards. (Of course the house was empty as usual.) Actually, I'm still not sure whether he was upset because they were there or because he wasn't included in the card game! Nevertheless, I suggested he just let them carry on and we'd go into the den and watch television. That suited him fine and he forgot all about it. Other times though, he wouldn't give up so easily and he would drive me almost crazy, wanting me to do something when there was nothing I could do.

Sometimes he would insist that he wanted to go home! Of course, as you know by now, that was one of his favourite topics. You couldn't tell him he was already home, as he would have convinced himself that home was somewhere else, so I'd have to humour him. By that time he'd forgotten his current address entirely, having regressed even further into the past, so whenever anyone would ask him where home was, he'd say London, England. He could even recite his home address in England, from when he was a little boy, and would insist that it was his present address. By then his Canadian address had completely ceased to exist in his memory. Sometimes he'd pack up all his belongings (usually an odd assortment of articles) in a bag, or even just in his arms, and ask me to call him a taxi to take him home.

At those times I'd say, "Well, if you'll wait until I'm finished (whatever I was doing), I'll take you home myself."

That would satisfy him for a short while but then he'd be after me again, constantly demanding to know when we were leaving. Then, when he could wait no longer, I would take him either for a walk or for a drive in the car, in either case ending up back at the house we'd just left.

Then I'd make a big issue out of saying "We're back home now! Isn't it nice to be home again?"—or something equally as exciting.

Interestingly enough this usually worked and he'd be quite content to be back home again—at least until the next time! Sometimes, if it happened during the day, we'd just go for a walk around the block, especially if the weather was nice (any excuse to give him some exercise) and it would also work as well. However, at one point he actually came to believe that there were two houses with the same furnishings and he was convinced that someone had stolen some of his furniture and pictures to put into the other house.

Another time he told me how he was selling chunks of beef to various people that day, but some of them had refused to pay him and he was upset. (I managed to restrain myself from asking, "Where's the beef?")

All I could do was commiserate with him and suggest he not sell to those people again. He actually seemed satisfied at that, which rather surprised me. Sometimes I think he was just happy that I took him seriously and answered his questions, instead of trying to argue him out of his notions, which never worked anyway!

Edwin enjoyed listening to me read to him every day and I tried to vary the selections. In the morning I would read from the newspapers but afternoons I'd choose poetry or a novel, something soothing. I'm sure he didn't follow most of the stories I read, but he seemed to enjoy the gentle tone of my voice, reacting to the cadence or rhythmic flow of sound. Sometimes he would doze off, only to rouse again if I stopped reading. One morning I was reading his horoscope, thinking he might get a kick out of it.

It said, "Romantic dry spell ends, Sagittarius."

Then I asked him what he thought of it, expecting him to smile or something.

"So Edwin," I asked, "what do you think of that?"

He replied, "Does that mean it's going to rain?"

Another evening he asked me, "Who runs this place?"

Then he went on to ask a number of questions including, "How do you fit into this scenario? Are you also a patient here? Do you have Alzheimer's too?" (Yes, he actually used the word!)

When the questions stopped, I tried to explain to him that I was his wife.

He looked crestfallen and said, "Of course, I should have known."

After that I walked into the living room and sat down. He followed me into the room, seating himself in front of me and proceeded to question me again.

"Who are you anyway?"

Once more I answered, "I'm your wife."

"No you're not!" he accused.

I assured him that I was his wife but he still insisted I was not, so I asked him his wife's name. He knew it was Marine or something like that, so I said "Marian?"

"Yes," he said, "Marian, that's her name, but you're not my wife, you're not Marian!"

At times like that I just felt sick to my stomach!

The next day Edwin had a terrible fall and it was a miracle he wasn't hurt. He just lost his balance and fell over backwards, crashing into the china cabinet. The doors flew open from the force of the impact and a lot of dishes went crashing down around him. He suffered huge red welts on his back, which had receded noticeably by that evening, but other than that he sustained no real injury. It always amazed me that he never broke any bones during his falls but for some reason he always seemed to be so relaxed when he fell, never tensing up or trying to stop himself from falling, that he'd come through relatively unscathed. He'd just let it happen, like someone who is inebriated or someone in a deep sleep. Maybe it was being so relaxed that prevented any serious damage—perhaps that was the key. In many cases, people sustain an injury through trying to avoid an accident, reacting to the danger by putting out their hands to stop themselves. In his case, having no fear of falling, or perhaps experiencing no real sense or awareness of danger, precluded his fighting against it, thus avoiding more serious injury. Whatever it was, I was grateful, because I know it sure scared me, every time it happened!

On Canada Day I had invited our neighbours, Pat and Bill, to come over for a barbecue on the patio. They had been so helpful and had treated us to dinner at their home on several occasions so I thought it would be nice to reciprocate in this way, as well as being a nice change for Edwin. Unfortunately he didn't see it that way. He knew they were coming but was surly and rude when they arrived. In fact he met them at the door, telling them right off that they couldn't stay because he had to go out. Usually he would use his social skills when among other people, especially ones with whom he felt comfortable, but not that day. They weren't sure what to think but they tried their best to draw him out of his mood and put him at ease. However, all afternoon he kept telling them they had to leave because he had to go for a CAT scan. The appointment had been set up two months previously and wasn't to take place for another two months but nothing would convince him that he shouldn't be going there right at that moment in time! When he'd get something into his head...well, you know by now!

Anyway, the entire afternoon was a disaster and I apologized profusely to our friends. However, I'm sure they understood, even though it was disappointing for all of us. At times he could be so good and well behaved but I could never plan on it. For that reason I could never have company over, except for very close friends, as I never knew what to expect and at times it could be extremely embarrassing—even humiliating.

That evening Edwin started in on the house again, asking, "What sort of place is this anyway?"

"It's our home," I answered. Then I asked, "Just who do you think I am?"

"Nurse Nightingale!" was his ready reply.

Later he asked, "Just how did you manage to get all the bric-a-brac over here?"

"It's always been here," I said.

His reply to that was to say, "There's obviously something I don't know!"

Most mornings Edwin would seem fairly normal, but as the day progressed, once again he would become confused and disorientated. Then would begin the pacing, the litany of weird questions and the strange, nonsensical conversations. It almost became a daily schedule. One day he was walking around looking for the bathroom, trying to get there by way of the front door.

Then he called me to ask, "Where is the key to the lavatory?"

He no longer used the word bathroom but had reverted to the word he'd always used back in England. Of course, there was no key and I finally had to go and show him where the bathroom was and how to use the toilet—without a key!

Later on he asked me again, what he was doing there in that place, so I explained once more that it was his home, where he'd lived for over 39 years.

"Does that mean I lived here when I was younger?" he asked.

I said, "Yes."

"But that's incredible!" he said, astounded. "How could I have lived here and not known it?"

How indeed! I thought to myself.

Then I asked him what his home address was.

He promptly replied, "One-O-Four Lexham Gardens, London W8."

"But what about Peace Drive?" I asked, quoting the address where we were currently living.

He replied, thoughtfully, "That rings a bell but I can't place it."

Later on he mentioned that he'd been away a long time and that a lot of things had changed during that time. Thinking he was referring to our time in Florida, I asked him where he'd been while he was away.

With no hesitation he answered, "Both in Sri Lanka (where he was stationed during the war) and in Canada."

He appeared to be under the illusion that he was back in London, England where he had lived as a boy. He was also convinced that other people lived in the home as well. When I denied that, he insisted there were four people in the living room at that very moment. One was (supposedly) playing the harp (of all instruments to choose) and two, a man and a woman, were playing bridge.

Some nights he would become quite amorous, wanting to have sex with me. Even now I find it embarrassing to speak of this, but I think it's necessary to cover this aspect of living with Alzheimer's as much as any other. Now each individual would have to handle that area of life in their own way, deciding ultimately what is best for them. For me, however, it was impossible! It was something I just couldn't face! First of all, how could he want to have sex with me, when to him, I was a total stranger, and not his wife? I found the whole scenario strange and uncomfortable, like sleeping with a stranger. I couldn't do it! Besides, Edwin had become like a child to me, ever since that fateful night on our way to Florida. I had to do everything for him, from bathing and dressing him, to wiping his bottom after he used the toilet. How then, could I possibly make love to him after doing all that? Perhaps if he had known me still, I might have felt differently about the situation, in fact I'm sure I would have, but as it was, he had become like a stranger to me, a trusting infant. It would have been like doing it with a child! It just seemed impossible for me and I felt humiliated each time he tried to initiate the act.

At first I would just refuse his advances, but that always ended in a big scene—just what I was trying to avoid! I'd cry over the problem, and even prayed about it, but I just didn't know how to handle the situation. Then one day I asked the specialist, thinking he might have some insight for me. However, he was no help at all.

When I told him, he just exclaimed, "You mean he can still do it?"

So much for help in that direction! I was totally embarrassed!

As I mentioned before, each care-giver has to do what's best for them and I certainly do not want to pass judgment on anyone. It's a very difficult subject at best, and I would never presume to tell anyone else how to handle it. However, I did find a solution that worked for me and I want to share it here, for the sake of those who are, perhaps, undergoing a similar dilemma. Whether it's of any help to others in their own situations remains to be seen, but I will relate it here, if only to give someone a smile.

It was always patently obvious when my husband wanted sex, as he'd tear off all his clothes before going to bed. I would then delay going to bed myself, as long as possible, hoping he would fall asleep, which he often did. Failing that, I would lie there passively when he touched me, and again, in time, he would eventually fall asleep, having forgotten his intentions by then. (Thank heavens for a short attention span.) The following morning, if he tried it again, I would respond to him as follows.

"Oh no, honey, I couldn't possibly do it again. You wore me out last night!"

"I did?" he'd say, grinning. "How was it?"

"Oh, it was wonderful!" I'd answer. "You were an animal!"

"I was?" he'd say, surprised. "I'm sorry I don't remember, but I'm glad you enjoyed it."

He would be quite happy at that, and inordinately pleased with himself, grinning from ear to ear. It actually worked too—every time—and the best part was...we were both happy!

As time wore on, the mornings started to get worse, becoming more like the afternoons and evenings. For a long while I had usually been able to count on him to be reasonable for that one part of the day and tried to schedule things that required his participation during those hours. However, that "prime time" gradually became shorter as the days progressed and by noon, if not before, he'd have started firing his usual barrage of questions, over and over again.

"What is the purpose of this place?"

"Why are they keeping me here?"

"Who runs this place?"

After cleaning up the lunch dishes one day, I was passing by Edwin's chair on the way to the kitchen. On an impulse I bent down to give him a light kiss on the back of his neck. He looked so shocked that I asked if he had minded my doing it.

"No I don't mind," he responded.

"I thought maybe you didn't like it?" I said.

"Oh no," he replied, "I'm just surprised, because the people that clear tables aren't usually so kind."

Then it was my turn to be shocked!

One night he was worse than usual; very upset and bound and determined he was leaving to go home.

"Why am I being kept in jail?" he demanded to know.

"What did I do wrong?"

"Why are you treating me this way?"

He became more and more agitated, convinced he was being held there against his will, not recognizing our home at all and claiming he had just gone there for an official paper of some sort and wanted to leave.

"Why are you holding me in jail?" he wailed.

"Why are you being so cruel to me?"

Finally, in desperation, I decided it was necessary to get him out of the house for a while. We were already undressed for bed but I dressed both of us again, calling my friend Alma to see if we could drop over for a short visit. I just couldn't handle him myself any more and knew we both had to get away from there, before things got out of hand. Alma was wonderful, caring and kind, and handled Edwin beautifully, acting more as a confidant to his alter persona. She treated us to coffee and her delicious cookies and was a great help in calming him down. In her own calm and soothing manner, she helped to explain to Edwin that he was living in his own home and had been there for over 39 years, while she herself lived just up the street from him. Poor Edwin, it was as though the fog had suddenly lifted, allowing him to see again and he became very contrite for what he'd put me through. He then talked about his days in the Royal Air Force, when he was required to obtain papers with his orders on them, before he could go anywhere. He also admitted that sometimes he would get things mixed up. (An understatement if ever there was one!)

I might just interject here to say that Edwin knew Alma, long before he knew me, as she had been a neighbour all the years he'd lived in that house. However, even though he did respond to her calming charms, he asked me later just who she was. He had no idea! In spite of that lack of recognition, though, I'm sure that he actually did recognize her on some sub-conscious level. He just didn't know it! Just as he didn't know who I was, but he understood, subconsciously too perhaps, that I was someone who loved him and cared for him, looking after him and caring for his needs. In fact, I was someone upon whom he depended for everything in his life.

The following evening at least we were not in jail again. Instead, by then the house had become a private boarding school in London, England! He had no idea who I was, as usual, only that I ran the school, and he subjected me to the usual barrage of questions:

"Have you worked here for a long time?"

"Long enough." I answered.

"Do you do all the work?"

"Yes, of course I do."

"Don't you have any maids?"

He was visibly shocked when I said no.

"You don't? But that's terrible!"

"We can't afford a maid."

"Do you get about the same number of people each day?"

"Yes, just you," I said, expecting a reaction to that.

He appeared to overlook my answer, asking instead,

"Has anyone showed an interest in the school since you worked here?"

"It's not a school," I tried telling him again.

"Have you traveled to many schools in your position?"

"No." I answered, resigned to the conversation.

Then he reverted to one of his regular questions, "Do any of the "old boys" know I'm back?"

Trying to change the subject, I commented on his new shoes.

He then said, "They were bought for me by a very loving lady."

"Who was the lady?" I asked.

"My wife," he answered.

"Where is your wife now?" I questioned.

There was a long silence before he replied, "That's a very good question. She's like you, flitting from one thing to another, always busy, always doing kind things. She was a loving lady. She was a grandmother. I like to think she's in heaven now. You met a good friend of hers the other night, the lady who entertained us. She lives just a few doors away." (He was referring to Alma.)

I wasn't sure why he thought I was dead, or at least in heaven, but wondered if he was, perhaps, thinking of his first wife, although she wasn't a grandmother like me. However, I realized he wasn't thinking of Trudy when he went on to say the following.

"My son's mother died too, a long time ago. She died of too much smoking."

That last part was all true. Once again I was amazed at the things he would remember and the sentiments he'd express, while still forgetting huge chunks of his life—like me for example! Sometimes it was all just unexplainable!

After dinner we went for a nice walk during which Edwin noticed the street signs. He expressed his surprise at the fact of my living so close to him, so I asked him where he lived. Once again he gave his full London address from childhood.

One day Edwin suddenly noticed the masses of red flowers in our front garden. They had been there for two months already, but that day he noticed them for the first time and was quite impressed.

That night he asked as usual, where he should sleep and I showed him to the bedroom again, commenting on the fact that we only had one bed.

"It looks like a very nice one too!" he replied enthusiastically.

I had to smile at that, it sounded so ludicrous, and especially since he was referring to a bed he'd slept in for so many, many years!

The following day he was having his usual daily panic, looking for his money, which he had moved from his wallet to his key case but was convinced had been stolen. I would show him where it was but ten minutes later he'd return with the same problem, over and over again. It would get so frustrating sometimes, that I'd think the only solution was to take all of it away from him. Eventually I knew it would come to that anyway, but until then I just kept trying to be patient. Every day there would be at least one major panic over something he couldn't find. Usually it involved items he had lost, but one day it was me he was looking for and he refused to go to bed until he found me. He'd declare, over and over, that he was looking for his wife, Marian, and he'd call my name. I kept answering, of course, but he wouldn't accept the fact that I was the right one. It was very depressing and frustrating as well, but mostly it just made me sad.

By that time Edwin was unable to do anything any more without step-by-step instructions and even then he had problems. When I asked him to get the cordless phone for me, after showing him to the den where the phone was always kept, he tried to bring the entire telephone, instead of just the handset, nearly ripping it out of the wall. Once he did the same thing with the TV set and managed to pull the wire right out of the wall, leaving the plug behind, still in the outlet. He was beginning to pose a real danger to himself, in many ways, and he bore constant watching.

Eventually he forgot how to eat a sandwich as well, his favourite food, and started eating it layer by layer. I tried to explain to him about picking up the whole sandwich to eat so he picked up the plate and all, nearly breaking his tooth when he tried to bite it! Then I had to show him how to pick up one section of the sandwich at a time, keeping both pieces of bread together.

The same thing occurred when I served him a hamburger. He ate the relish and catsup off the top. Then he commented, "Good dinner!"

After enjoying lunch one day, Edwin turned to me, making the following remark.

"I take it the Central Authority pays for all this food?"

On more than one occasion he'd imagine he was living in a boarding school. (That obviously went back to his younger days in England.) Also, as mentioned previously, several times he'd ask me if the "old boys" knew he was back yet. (Whoever the "old boys"' might be. No doubt his buddies from London.) At those times he'd think I was the headmistress of the boarding school and would marvel at all the work I would do. Then when I'd start cooking dinner, he'd question why I had to do everything. Why didn't I have servants to do it? When I'd say I couldn't afford it, he'd insist that we must do something about that! (Unfortunately, he never did!)

At other times he'd be convinced that I was the cook and ask where everybody else had gone. Then again, he'd think I was the gardener, or the doctor, or the chauffeur, and so forth. After I cut my hair short, something more manageable and less time-consuming, since I couldn't leave him alone for the length of time it took to wash and curl it, he'd refer to me as "the boy." Then again, he'd ask where the boy had gone. Sometimes as well, he'd be looking for his wife. However, when I'd answer him, trying to assure him that I was there, he'd insist that I wasn't his wife. Then I'd ask him what his wife's name was. He'd fumble about a bit and then say, Marine, or something like that. Again I'd question him, asking if her name was

Marian? When he'd reply to the affirmative, I'd tell him again that I was Marian, his wife, but he'd still insist I wasn't the one.

Sometimes I'd have an inspiration and say to him, "Maybe you mean Trudy." Since she was his first wife, who had died some years before and she dated back to his days in the Air Force, it made sense to me that he would remember her before me. With his loss of recent memory he seemed to be living more and more in the past anyway, so I thought maybe that was the answer. However, he'd always deny even knowing a Trudy and insist again that his wife's name was Marine, or something like that. I even tried showing him a photograph of Trudy, on several occasions, but there was never any recognition whatsoever.

How sad to think that an entire lifetime had been wiped away in one swift stroke. From now on I shall always savour my memories, both good and bad, realizing that everything in life has a purpose, and nothing is ever lost if we can learn from it. By the same reasoning, everyone is brought into our lives for a reason and to fulfill a certain need at that time. Memories become sweeter when we grasp that truth, and even heartaches are tempered by the passing of time, leaving us with only the memories of the good times we shared, rather than the pain. Through all those years of living with Alzheimer's, I learned to cherish my memories and enjoy each new day as a gift from God. Because life has no guarantees, we need to "seize the moment" and let the years take care of themselves. There is a verse in the King James version of the Bible that I thought about a lot those days. It is found in Deuteronomy 33:25 and reads as follows:

As thy days, so shall thy strength be.

Simply translated, it just means that God will give us the strength we need, *when* we need it! I don't have the strength today to face tomorrow, but when tomorrow becomes today, God will provide the strength I need to face that day and to carry on, one day at a time, one step at a time!

Home Is Just a State of Mind

Many times while we were in Florida, Edwin would bring up the subject of his home, but even at that time, home did not evoke pictures of our house in Canada. It referred instead to his home in London, England as a child.

He'd express concern, saying, "I hope my son isn't staying at my home in Kensington, London, just for something to do."

I would try to explain to him that he no longer lived in England, to which he would respond by asking where he did live now, if not in London. When we finally did arrive back to our home in Canada, he still didn't recognize it, even though he'd lived there for so long. In fact, shortly after arriving home I came across him packing his razor and slippers in his camera bag.

"What are you doing?" I asked him.

"It's time for me to leave this library," he answered, "so I'm getting ready to go home."

Later that same day I found him putting on his shoes, again getting ready to leave, convinced that we were not in the same house we'd been in earlier that day. In other words, that location meant nothing to him. His home for over 39 years had ceased to exist, at least in his mind.

When I called Edwin for lunch one day he asked, "Are there any rules regarding what I can eat, and quantities, that sort of thing?"

I assured him he could have whatever he wanted and however much he desired, as it was his home.

He then commented, "I wonder who lived here before?"

I told him, "No one else lived here before you. You bought the place new, even before they'd finished building it."

He then asked, "Did my father or mother live here?"

I finally managed to divert his train of thought by asking him to tell me about his mother and father.

During lunch he mentioned his upcoming CAT scan again, saying, "I don't understand why I had to come here for it, when they must have hospitals with all the necessary equipment?"

I said, "You *are* going to the hospital to have it done."

"You mean they're not going to do it here?" he asked.

"Right!" I answered.

"Then why did I have to come here?" he asked.

"Because you live here," I replied. "This is your home!"

A few minutes later he started in again, commenting, "I still don't understand why they put all that expensive (CAT scan) equipment in here though."

"They didn't!" I said.

"Who did then?"

"Nobody did! It's not in here!" I was getting a little exasperated by that time.

"Where did you learn all this?" he asked.

"All what?" I wanted to know.

"The business you're in now," he replied, equally exasperated. "Did you work in a hospital?"

"No, I didn't."

"How long have you been working here?"

"A long time."

"How did you get the job? You must have had certain qualifications to get it."

"I married you!" I answered.

That shut him up for a few minutes before he commented, "You certainly do come up with some astounding things!"

"Well," I said, "who am I then?"

"Obviously you must be somebody, or you wouldn't be qualified to work here," he replied, "but just who you are I can't figure out."

After lunch he gave me twenty dollars to cover his bill for the meal!

When he finally did go for his long-awaited CAT scan it went very well indeed. All his worrying was for nothing. Of course, then we had to wait a couple of weeks for the results. However, Edwin figured that since they told us nothing at the hospital, it must mean that he was fine and nothing was wrong with him. He was convinced by then that he was completely healed. (If only that had been true!) In fact, when his son phoned to see how the CAT scan had gone, Edwin told him that he was all better now, sounding almost normal on the phone too. I think he was just relieved to have it over with. Obviously it had been preying on his mind for some time. Anyway, even though he sounded quite normal on the phone, after talking to his son, Edwin thanked me for having let him know where he was. He seemed very surprised that his son had been able to locate him in the first place, since he wasn't at home. His comment obviously indicated his conviction that he was living somewhere else himself, other than in his own house.

We arrived home from another of Edwin's medical appointments one day during a heavy rainfall. I hurried into the house, thinking Edwin was right behind me, but when I looked back he was still standing outside getting soaked.

"Come in! Come in!" I called, signalling with my arm.

He then yelled back to say, "Why would I want to go in there?"

"Because you live here!" I answered.

He just said, "Oh!" and came on in.

I then hung up my jacket and turned to get his, but

he was busily engaged in trying to hang his hat (a tweed fedora) on a hanger.

I really had thought that after 39 years in the same location, Edwin would be more comfortable there, but it just didn't seem to make any difference. I finally had to put up signs all over the house, just as I had done in Florida, indicating where everything was so he could find his way around. I realized even then that it wouldn't matter where he lived anymore. No place would ever be "home" to him. Not any more.

As much as possible I tried to maintain some semblance of a comfortable, homey atmosphere for my husband. To achieve this I would use the good china for dinner, serving the meal at the dining room table, rather than in the kitchen, and enhancing the atmosphere with music and candlelight or flowers. Other times I'd plan a picnic in the back yard on a beautiful summer day, or sit cosily beside him in the evening watching the television, or read to him while soft music played on the stereo. It really didn't matter what I read to him, since he couldn't understand what I was reading anyway, but the sound of my voice was soothing to him. He couldn't follow anything on the television, but he liked the pictures (sometimes) and he enjoyed sitting beside me on the love seat. In fact, even in regard to the fancy meals I prepared, it seemed to me that he could hardly taste what he was eating anymore, since that part of his brain, the area that controls the ability to taste, appeared to have been affected as well, but he enjoyed the atmosphere of peace induced by a few candles and some quiet background music. Maybe I was trying to convince myself that everything was normal as well—I really don't know—but whatever my reasoning or subconscious motives, all these things helped to create an aura of peaceful, loving, security; something desperately needed in the frightening, shadowy world of Alzheimer's, and I don't regret any of the effort I expended on such endeavours.

As well, whenever possible, I'd set him tasks to perform, within the scope of his ability and expertise, in order to give him a sense of worth. One of the tasks I'd assign him would be to blow out the candles after dinner in the evening. Of course I'd have to instruct him each time, but that was a normal occurrence for me by then. However, invariably, following my instructions he'd blow out one candle only before leaving the table. On discovering the others still burning, I'd call him back to finish the job.

Then he would promptly reply, "Oh, I didn't know you wanted me to blow out the candles."

It was useless to point out that yes, he did know, since he had already blown out the first candle, because by then he'd have forgotten having done it at all. In fact, after blowing out the first candle he would forget what he was supposed to be doing—or was doing—thus explaining why he'd left the others lit. In other words, his short-term memory was becoming extremely short-term, so much so in fact, that he would forget what he was doing in the middle of doing it!

It was the same with dressing in the morning. I'd get him started, laying out his clothes for the day and encouraging him to do it himself as much as possible. However, halfway through the job he'd start to undress again. He could never remember if he was supposed to be dressing or undressing or if it was time to get up or time to go to bed. At night it was a repeat performance—except backwards. Eventually, of course, he was not able to do anything for himself at all any more and I had to do everything for him, from dressing him, to bathing him, shaving him and wiping his bottom, not to mention all the other unpleasant tasks that one is required to perform on a daily basis. In other words, it was like having a young child again—only a very large one!

One evening Edwin was particularly upset and angry with the world in general, so much so, that when I "gently" tossed his key case and wallet into the top drawer of his dresser for the night, he reacted rather violently, literally jumping on me and yelling in my ear.

"Don't you dare throw my things around!"

Of course I apologized immediately, even if it wasn't deliberate, but the incident really scared me. I'd never seen him looking so angry and intense and the way he lunged at me seemed so menacing. I decided it was time I left his room for a while—and quickly! Later on, after I'd changed into my nightgown, he came to me, very apologetic and insisted on taking me out for a drink to make up for his behaviour. He just would not take no for an answer, and rather than aggravate him further, I agreed. I changed my clothes, again, and took him in the car to the Red Lobster, where I knew they offered fancy "virgin" drinks. Actually, he really enjoyed the outing and was good company. We sat at the bar enjoying our fruit drinks while I explained to him what "virgin" drinks were. (That means no alcohol, for the uninitiated!) He found them very tasty and was quite impressed.

Before leaving the restaurant he turned to me and said, "You know, that's the first virgin I've ever had!"

I doubt that he realized he'd made a joke, or even how funny it was, but I had to laugh and he laughed along with me, unaware of the humour but enjoying the camaraderie.

I treasured that little interlude as one of our special moments together, for the next day it was back to normal. Edwin was absolutely "off-the-wall" for most of the day. He tried leaving home several times, the first attempt being with his camera case in a large plastic bag. He waited until I was in the bathroom and then took off. I caught up to him heading around the corner of the street, so I joined him, walking around the entire block, hoping to wear him out. No such luck though, as he made another attempt at leaving that same day. That one took him out the back door and around the side of the house, where I found him before he managed to get away. However, that time he refused to go back into the house with me so I finally walked him over to Alma's place for a short visit. Fortunately she was home and welcomed us, as always, with open arms. After that visit he was quite willing to go home again, having enjoyed the interlude and forgotten his original intentions.

In the evening, while I was busy cooking hamburgers on the barbecue, he took off again, this time to Pat and Bill's house with his camera bag. He told them he wanted to leave his camera there as I was trying to steal it from him. Actually, it wasn't such a bad idea to leave it there, I thought, at least for a while, since out of sight could also prove out of mind, at least I hoped that might be the case. After dinner he tried once more to leave the house, but that time I had already set the alarm so was alerted instantly. I dreaded the coming night, knowing it would probably be more of the same.

I wasn't disappointed!

After that particular day, the doctor doubled Edwin's medication, as well as putting him on a sleeping pill. He never wanted to sleep anymore and wouldn't even doze during the day at all either. Honestly, I don't know where he got all his energy. I sure could have used some of it myself. By then I was drained and exhausted. In fact, I went to visit the doctor myself after that, hoping he could offer some suggestions in handling Edwin, but he was more concerned with my well-being.

He lectured me in no uncertain terms, saying, "It's about time you got off this train going nowhere, and get Edwin established in a special care unit where they can help him." He also went on to explain, "The earlier dementia patients go into a nursing facility, the better they settle in, and waiting too long can also be detrimental, as often they never really adjust to the change."

What he said made sense, I knew, but I just could not bring myself to make such a decision. I kept thinking about how I would feel if it were myself, and I couldn't do it. Edwin needed me! How could I ever put him into a nursing home? It was unthinkable! Later maybe, but not now, not yet!

And so we carried on!

So much for the new sleeping pills! That night, after taking his new pill, Edwin was up and down all night, searching through his drawers, knocking things over and pulling the cushions off the couches in the living room and den. The place looked like a disaster area in the morning, but the final straw was when Edwin questioned me as to why I kept the place in such a mess! Why indeed? (Patience! Patience!)

One morning when I took Edwin to the Day Program, the workers met us at the door on our arrival and asked me, in front of Edwin, if we could bring his camera to the program the next time. Having no idea of the "history of frustration" behind his camera, they thought it might be a great idea, since Edwin had been a photographer and could possibly talk to the others about his interest in photography. Of course, they were unaware of the Pandora's Box which any allusion to the word "camera" could open, but they soon found out to their dismay! As soon as he heard their request, Edwin was off! It triggered one of his fits of pique, which ultimately exploded into a full blown, vitriolic rage, as he demanded to know where his camera was! What had they done with it? Who had stolen it? The regular drill!

I tried desperately to calm him down, as did the others, but to no avail. The damage had been done and they were now subjected to the Edwin I saw almost every night at home. I'm sure they were shocked, but I'm also sure that this wasn't the first time they had seen such a transformation in an Alzheimer's patient. Working with these people every day as they did, they'd probably seen a lot worse. However, that knowledge didn't help me in swallowing my embarrassment and my own dismay at his behaviour. He was adamant in refusing to stay at the centre, claiming instead that he needed to go to the "hotel" to find his camera. It took three workers to corner him, diverting his attention, while another one hauled me out of there and sent me home. I was averse to going but they insisted I should leave so I did, burning up with humiliation but worried for them as well. What was going to happen next, I wondered? He was becoming embarrassingly bellicose, quarrelsome and hostile, not to mention frightening, and I wondered just how much longer I'd be able to handle him if he were to continue on like that. It was all very worrying, to say the least!

That evening when I picked him up he was still fuming, calling the workers all sorts of terrible names, ranting and raving, and accusing them of lying to him. I was afraid that if his aggressive behaviour continued, they would have to exclude him from the Day Care Centre, a concern that worried me constantly by then.

By that time he was doing so many strange and crazy things that I hardly know what to recount. At bedtime I found him with one leg in the arm of his kimono. He had inserted his leg into the wrist end of the housecoat and pulled it all the way up. When I arrived on the scene, he was busily trying to insert the other leg into the second armhole and had become totally tangled in the process. Needless to say, I had a terrible time trying to remove the garment as it was tightly lodged on his person.

The following day I took him for a walk in the park. It was a lovely day and I felt the fresh air and exercise would do us both some good. He enjoyed it, to an extent, but was constantly on the lookout for, and fearful of "kids with long knives," and also of "people who might punch him with their elbows." Honestly, it seemed like he was becoming fearful of everything and everybody by then, while developing more aggressively hostile behaviour himself.

The next morning I went out for my early morning walk as usual. However, that day Edwin did not await my return, safely asleep in his bed, as was his normal routine. That day he awoke early and decided to go for a walk himself, looking for me. I met him half way up the street, resolutely walking towards me, wearing only his undershirt and shorts! He would have marched right on past me too, as there was no recognition on his part, but I took his hand and walked him back home. I was just grateful that most of our neighbours were not early risers—at least not *that* early!

Driving in the car one day, with Edwin beside me in the front seat, I narrowly averted an accident as he suddenly grabbed my wrist and would not let go. His grip was like a vice as I tried to free my arm and I was thoroughly alarmed. I was in the process of navigating a turn and couldn't manage it without both hands on the steering wheel but he refused to release his grasp. I actually had to fight him off, hitting his arm and even yelling at him before he released me. It was a frightening situation, which could easily have resulted in an accident, but Edwin had no concept of what he'd done or the danger of his actions. However, he was mad at me for having yelled at him and pouted the rest of the morning. That wasn't the first time he'd done that sort of thing, but it was the most frightening. Actually, he was becoming a real threat to safety in the car, engendering yet another concern about this aspect of his behaviour and causing me to wonder just how long it would be before something tragic occurred.

All those incidents were beginning to add up to a serious threat to our safety, to his safety, and for the future. How much longer would I be able to control him? How much longer before his actions precipitated a dangerous situation, a serious accident, or something equally tragic? I didn't know the answer but I dreaded the future, as my own life seemed to be careening out of control, and fearful apprehension took hold of me, as the road ahead loomed frightening and ominous!

As his condition rapidly deteriorated, I realized that in due time I was going to have to put him into a nursing home, as I could not give him such intensive care for-ever. As the saying goes: *They bury the caregivers*, and already I sensed that my health was sliding downhill, as I was losing weight and going without sufficient sleep. Still I determined to keep him at home as long as I pos-sibly could. I felt he just wasn't ready for a nursing home yet, nor was I ready to give him up! Several of his doc-tors were encouraging me to make the move and sug-gested that I needed to get his name on the waiting list for a long-term care facility, as sometimes the wait, espe-cially for the more desirable homes, could be long. I knew they were right but I just couldn't bring myself to acknowledge it, much less do something about it. And so I continued to persevere, but the struggle continually grew more difficult until, finally, the situation was taken out of my hands and the choice was no longer mine to make. Edwin had been admitted to the hospital, in dire straits mentally, and now required full-time medical care. The doctors would no longer allow him to return home with me, stipulating that he must stay in the hos-pital until he could be admitted to a nursing home.

The time had come!

The day I had long dreaded had arrived! Determined to take him to the nursing home myself, rather than subject him to being transported by ambu-lance, I refused the hospital's offer to deliver him to his new residence, resigned to doing the job myself. I didn't want him to feel that he was just going to be dumped there, nor did I want the transition to be too traumatic for him. Thus, on the appointed day, I arrived at the hospital with his suitcase and belongings, ready to drive him to his *new home*.

That time I had taken the doctor's advice and said nothing to Edwin about the move ahead of time. I knew from past experience that they were right, of course, as any time I spoke to him about coming events, he would begin to obsess over the occasion. Whether negatively or positively, it really didn't matter, he would just not let the subject drop, and would drive me crazy with wanting to know when he was going or what day it was going to happen. Also, in that particular case, I knew the thought of moving would have created far too much turmoil in his mind.

Thus I waited for the day to arrive and said simply, and clearly, "Come on Edwin, we're going home!"

He came along happily, complacently even, and almost eagerly, while I felt terribly guilty about misleading him, thinking he'd figure we were going to our house, but forgetting, of course, that in his mind our real "home" no longer existed.

If he was surprised at this new place called "home," he didn't show it. Much to my amazement and relief, he just accepted it as normal, without question, and began to settle in. I had already gone to the nursing home with Alma the day before, having paid for an extra day in order to decorate his room and make it "homey" for him, hanging pictures and dressing it up, to make it as comfortable and cozy as possible. I wanted to have it completely finished before bringing him over and moving him in so, hopefully, his first impression would be positive. I'd brought a nice dresser, his easy chair and ottoman from home, his own pillows and quilt, and a television set, as well as a few other things to make him feel at home. The room looked quite pleasant and inviting and I hoped he would be pleased, but I was still very nervous about his reaction to the move. In fact, I was so concerned, that the night before the transfer I was unable to sleep at all for thinking about it. However, all my worrying was totally unnecessary. As it turned out, I was the only one who was upset! Edwin accepted his new accommodations with no hassle whatsoever. He just took everything in his stride and offered no objections at all. I think his weeks in the hospital must have helped a lot, but even so, I was amazed at his reaction—or should I say, lack of negative reactions—to the situation. I had expected anything but that! In fact, shortly after his arrival, he became convinced that this was the same place where he used to live when he first came to Canada over forty years ago. I didn't try to dissuade him nor did I attempt to explain that this building was only six years old so it couldn't possibly be the same one. I was just relieved at his calm acceptance of the place and breathed a sigh of relief. He was at home there, wherever that might be, surrounded by his own things and comfortable with them. I guess it really is true, that old saying, "Home is just a state of mind!"

I took further comfort in the fact that my husband readily settled into the home, rather quickly and virtually painlessly. Actually, it took *me* far longer to adjust to the idea and to get over the feelings of guilt and inadequacy, fearing that I had failed him in some

way. However, his ready acceptance of his new surroundings affirmed for me other aspects of living with
Alzheimer's, more positive features of the disease (if I
can call anything positive about Alzheimer's). As we
know, Alzheimer's patients experience the ultimate of
living in, or for, the moment. They still have definition
as a person, but without a past. By this interpretation,
living in their own familiar homes, surrounded by
their old lives, which they cannot remember, only
increases the anxiety and frustration of trying to
remember, whereas life is simplified for them in the
nursing home. The feeling of familiarity is gone and
they are no longer confronted with the compulsion, or
pressure, of trying to remember things that are already
lost to them. In fact, that is also one of the reasons
medical specialists of the disease recommend early
placement, as opposed to waiting too long. Since the
patient tends to settle in more readily and easily when
they enter the nursing home environment before
becoming too used to their personal care-giver
catering to all their needs and wishes, the break is also
cleaner. Those who wait too long find that the patient
becomes used to having his own servant, as it were,
day and night. They may not remember who we are
but they do know we're there for them exclusively
and, like children, they do know how to take advantage of the situation, even to the extent of throwing
tantrums when they don't get their own way. Thus we,
the care-givers, end up exhausted and spent, devoting
24 hours a day trying to care for one person, and still
feeling inadequate, convinced somehow that we're

missing the mark in actually meeting the real needs of our patient. I know now that I was not alone in feeling that way but it still didn't make it any easier. It's a fine line and a difficult decision at best, and I'm afraid it shall always be thus. However, ultimately it has to come down to one very basic question.

"What is best for the patient?"

Not, "How do *I* feel about it?"

Not, "What is best for *me?*"

Not, "What is best for *my* peace of mind?"

Indeed, what is best for your loved one is not always what is best for you, or for your conscience—quite the contrary! No one would want to see a loved one suffer more than necessary, yet by hanging on we often accomplish just that. It's probably one of the hardest lessons we'll ever have to learn in life, but we need to know when to let go, when to learn for ourselves that *home is just a state of mind!*

Nights and Daze

CHAPTER 13

I should back up at this point and describe the events that led to my husband's admission to a nursing home, in spite of all my protestations to the contrary. His condition had been rapidly deteriorating and I was becoming more and more concerned, as well for myself as for my husband. Having lost so much weight and so much sleep because of having to care for him increasing hours of the day and night, I wondered how much longer I would be able to carry on without breaking down myself. Long before that stage, determined to try and get more rest, I had already curtailed any outside or personal activities, but even that wasn't enough.

How many more sleepless nights could I take? I would ask myself that question again and again, as wearily each night I followed Edwin from room to room, trying in vain to calm him down and get him back to bed.

"Let me give you a pill," I offered, for the third or fourth time one night. "It will help to settle you down."

"I don't want a pill!" he shouted over and over again.

"But it will help you to feel better," I tried again.

"Why are you trying to give me a pill?" he demanded. "Are you trying to poison me? What's in it, strychnine?"

Totally frustrated by that time, I replied, "No, its not strychnine, but only because I don't have any!"

I was so angry and upset by his determined efforts to thwart me at every turn, and bone weary from repeated nights such as that one, I finally lost my temper. However, as soon as I'd said it, I was sorry and tried to be loving and tender again, even apologizing to him for getting angry, but now, adding to my already heavy burden, was the feeling of guilt for my flare of temper. I'd failed again! I felt terrible!

"He's not responsible for his actions," I'd say in my head, having to remind myself yet again, trying to control my temper and trying to temper my frustration. He doesn't know what he's doing. My only comfort, in trying to assuage my feelings of failure and guilt, was the knowledge that tomorrow he wouldn't remember any of it and I could start all over again, trying to do it right! In a sense, the terrible, short-term memory loss, endemic to Alzheimer's disease, was also a blessing in a way, as each new day presented a fresh start—for both of us—a new opportunity to try again. No hangovers of guilt for me or recrimination on his part, but a complete new beginning—a clean slate as it were. The failures of yesterday were behind me; he would have forgotten about them entirely (if only I could) so he harboured no resentment for any uncharitable reactions I might have expressed the previous day. It reminded me of a movie I saw some time ago, called *Groundhog Day,* where each day the fellow got to start all over again until he finally got it right. I hoped that some day I could get it right too. Meanwhile I desperately tried to learn from my mistakes, so as not to repeat them, and I constantly prayed for patience and understanding in dealing with my husband.

Throughout those long nights he would march from room to room, searching for things, finding them, and then hiding them again in new, ingenious locations, as before, but with much more urgency and compulsion driving him on, robbing him also of much needed rest and sleep. The situation was definitely declining, getting much worse, and he was becoming more and more agitated with each passing night, spending more time pacing than in the past. Other nights he'd dress (and undress) himself, sometimes becoming hopelessly entangled in what he was trying to put on or remove. It was terribly frustrating for me as well, for I'd become so tired but wasn't able to go to bed myself. In fact, I didn't dare to go to sleep, fearing that Edwin might injure himself in his agitation, so as long as he was awake I needed to be there for him. Whatever he was feeling during those nocturnal sessions, it was equally frustrating for him I'm sure, as he was totally confused and didn't quite know himself, just what he wanted or was trying to do. If he did know, however briefly, during flashes of cognitive activity, it would soon be lost again, leaving him even more confused and vulnerable than before.

Sometimes he'd put on a shoe and then pull a sock on over the shoe. If it wouldn't fit, he'd become extremely frustrated and angry. Other times he'd try to put on his dressing gown, very carefully inserting his legs through the arm holes, then wondering why it was so hard to walk. One evening he put both legs into one arm of his kimono and I had an awful time trying to extricate him. Layering clothes was also one of his favourite activities, long before layering was popular, and he'd put on two or three shirts and two pairs of trousers with his underwear on top, or worn as a scarf. Once he even put on his undershirt around his hips, wearing it like a miniskirt, topping off his "ensemble" with a pair of long-legged Jockey shorts draped around his shoulders and another pair doubling as a handkerchief. Very inventive! (One morning I found him dressed like that in the Nursing home, happily strolling up and down the corridors, complete with one bare foot, while the other foot wore a shoe with a sock pulled over the shoe. The nurses were very embarrassed and apologetic about my finding him in this condition but I hastened to assure them that I was quite used to it and understood.)

Sometimes it's best to let them do their own thing rather than try to fight with them. When they want to do something for themselves it's better to let them, no matter what the outcome, as long as it's not dangerous, of course. Very often, coming back later will result in their allowing you then to fix them up properly, after they've had their show of independence. They seem to have their own schedule! I know Edwin certainly did! Forcing the issue would just aggravate him and often lead to violence. In fact, one of the nurses at the home found this out for herself, to her detriment. My husband was not a big man, nor was he of a violent nature normally, but with the Alzheimer's he would often fight for his own way. In this case the nurse was trying to get him dressed properly and he did not want to comply. When she tried to force the issue, he actually threw her against the wall, breaking his own eyeglasses in the ensuing struggle. Now one might be tempted to sympathize with the nurse, but bear one fact in mind. She was twice the size of my husband!

Yes, even a gentle man can invoke super-human strength when pushed too far. I too learned this the hard way!

One night, Edwin's normal nocturnal activities escalated into a nightmare from which there was no turning back! That night he went on a rampage, destroying everything in sight and even attacking me, almost breaking my arm. It all started just after we'd retired for the night. I was exhausted and had begun to doze off when he suddenly sat up, insisting he wanted to check his wallet, even though he'd already done so at least three times earlier. He got out of bed and turned on the lights but couldn't find the wallet, so I had to get up and show him where it was in his bureau drawer. He then picked up his sunglasses, which were also in the drawer, and shoved them into the pocket of his pyjamas, heading back to bed. I then suggested he remove the sunglasses from his pocket, as they would break if he wore them to bed.

That was all it took!

That simple comment became the trigger, and he flew into a complete rage, accusing me of "threatening to break his glasses!"

It just took off from there and he started to rail at me, accusing me of all manner of atrocities, from stealing his clothes to things I wouldn't even mention. He ranted and raved, pacing the floor and shouting obscenities, some of which I had never heard before— and that was just the beginning! That night his antics were even crazier than usual. While doing his rounds of marching from room to room, searching, hunting, hiding items, then searching again, things finally came to a head as his insupportable insanity reached an all time high. He'd been pacing for hours and I was afraid he was going to harm himself in his agitation if he didn't calm down, but he was like a wild animal in captivity. I was dead tired, and desperate to get the situation under control, but it proved impossible and I found myself simply unable to endure any more. I was so tired my entire body just threatened to shut down and I knew I had to get some rest before I became ill myself. I'd answered his incessant questions over and over and over again and now, having followed him from room to room and back to the bedroom, I finally made my declaration.

"That's it!" I said. "I can't take any more! I've got to get some sleep. I'm going to the living room."

So saying, I quickly grabbed my pillow from the bed, prepared to go to the other room and lie down, before I collapsed with fatigue. However, when I tried to walk out the door, Edwin started yelling and screaming at me, claiming that those were his pillows and that I couldn't steal his bedding and get away with it! He then lunged at me like a madman, grabbing my arm and screaming that I was "trying to steal his linens." The strength of his grip was phenomenal and I was totally surprised and overwhelmed. His hands were like a vise, hard and painful, and I thought for sure he'd break my wrist! His face was contorted in anger and his eyes looked wild and crazed. I can't begin to describe my fear at that moment, but I was in complete shock! My gentle, loving husband, the one who needed me and depended on me; the one I'd been desperately trying to protect all these months and shield from the cruel world; the one I loved above all else, had now become this wild, uncontrollable, crazy lunatic and turned on me! My heart began to beat erratically in my chest and panic threatened to engulf me as I struggled vainly to free myself and to escape the pain of his iron grip. In spite of my fear, I tried to talk soothingly to him, looking him in the eye, as all the books suggested, telling him that everything was all right, but even as I talked, his agitation grew and I began to fear for my life. Finally, with one last painful thrust I managed to wrench my arm out of his grasp and I fled to the living room in terror.

The room was dark, and since Edwin normally avoided dark places, I took a chance and lay down on the couch, although "cowering" would describe my actions more aptly. Flattening myself down into the cushions, I lay there in the dark, stiff but still, hardly daring to breathe, much less move, and afraid to close my eyes lest he sneak up on me in the darkness, despite his usual aversion to darkened rooms.

Edwin continued on his rampage, pacing the floors, marching from room to room, constantly busy, rattling drawers, emptying their contents on to the floor, pulling the bedding off the bed, marching into the den, tossing the cushions off the love seat, dumping the garbage cans, pulling his clothing out of the closet, tearing things apart, rustling papers and shuffling to and fro. He also wrapped a variety of his possessions in Kleenex, hiding them in rather unique locations, which I discovered the following day; tore down all my signs about the house, and proceeded to put on various and sundry pieces of apparel over his pyjamas. It was totally bizarre! He looked like a clown, wearing his weird concoction of clothing and marching about the house but—unlike his nemesis—he was not funny!

Meanwhile, I continued to lie there in the darkness on the couch, tense and fearful, eyes wide open, watching his progress from room to room; including several forays into the living room itself, where he'd walk right up to the couch I was lying on and just stand there for a while, before moving away again, to resume his destruction of the other rooms. I have no idea if he realized I was there or not, as I remained stiff and silent, even holding my breath, while he was standing in front of me, afraid to move or acknowledge his presence, but he did return several times during that long night and each time I would await the attack that, thankfully, never came. Each time he would just stand there looking down at me, but I don't think really seeing me, and then he'd move away once more, only to return again some time later and do the same thing.

Each time he came I'd go tense with fear, terribly afraid of what he might do to me in his extremely agitated state of mind; feeling alone and scared with nowhere to turn and no one to help me. I have never felt so alone, so vulnerable, as I did that night! I desperately needed help but there was no one to call. After all, who in the world could you call in the middle of the night? Thus I remained until the early hours of the morning, when Edwin finally wore himself out and crawled on top of his tumbled, dishevelled bed, falling immediately into an exhausted and sound sleep.

Even then I waited, wanting to be sure that he really was sleeping, before I dared to move, before I could make myself leave the refuge of my couch.

The next morning I saw all the evidence of his rampage and I might have laughed, had I not been so overwrought from the terror of that long night. The bedroom and his den were in a shambles, with shelves and drawers emptied and overturned, and clothing pulled from the closets, lying everywhere in disarray. Things were knocked off the shelves and strewn about the rooms, and even the garbage cans were full, but not with garbage. It looked like the aftermath of a cyclone and I stared in awe at his handiwork. At this point he himself was sleeping soundly, in the midst of the turmoil, blissfully unaware of the chaos he had created.

I knew that he would sleep for some time after such a strenuous night, but by then I was too upset to consider sleeping myself, so I decided to go for a walk and think things through. The long night had taken its toll and I was a nervous wreck. I had to get outside, to get some fresh air and somehow calm my frazzled nerves. I couldn't stop shaking and my heart kept beating in staccato time. I couldn't take much more and I knew I was ready to break, but I just didn't know what to do.

What could I do?

On returning from my walk, I noticed that Alma's door was open, our silent signal that guests were welcome, and desperately needing to talk to someone, I stopped in. As always she welcomed me warmly and put on the coffee pot. However, also extremely perceptive, she realized immediately that something was very wrong with me, something more than usual, and she encouraged me to talk about it. Once I began though, I couldn't stop, and the whole, frightening story of the previous night's experience tumbled from my lips as my tears flowed freely. Never one to avoid truths, no matter how painful, she impressed on me the need to get help, emphasizing the fact that I could not go on this way, losing sleep, losing weight and endangering my own life as well as Edwin.

I knew she was right but I guess I just needed to hear it from someone else. At her insistence, that same day, I phoned for an emergency appointment and took my husband to see the psychiatrist he had been referred to at the hospital. (While there, I also had my arm checked out, as it was still very painful. Fortunately it was not broken, but it was badly sprained and I was required to wear a brace on it for a few weeks until it healed.)

When confronted by the doctor with his actions of the night before, Edwin was clearly shocked.

"I would never hurt my wife," he avowed. "I love her. She's so good to me; why would I want to hurt her?"

He was terribly upset, but *had no memory whatsoever* of the previous night's activities, unbelievable as it might seem.

Meanwhile, I had hoped the doctor could prescribe some other medication for Edwin, that would help him through this, but that was not the case and at length the Doctor insisted that Edwin be placed in the hospital for assessment. Of course I objected strongly, for my husband's sake, but I was overruled, and he was admitted, there and then, to the psychiatric ward of the hospital. I realized the doctor was probably right, of course, but it still didn't make it any easier to accept, and after seeing him to his room, I went home in tears, to pack a suitcase for him, feeling that I had failed him somehow, in not being able to prevent the inevitable. The hospital made me take home all of his clothes, as they wanted him in hospital attire, so as to prevent his wandering away. He also had to wear a special bracelet, which would signal the office if he should try to exit the floor.

The next two weeks saw me spending each afternoon and evening at the hospital. (Visitors were not allowed in the morning as that time was used for various therapies and procedures.) Edwin's son also came most afternoons after work, and I know Edwin appreciated his visits, even though he was less than responsive. One afternoon while I was visiting him, Edwin kept looking out the window from his room, which overlooked several hydro towers and a large, white water tower.

He commented, "See the many walkie-talkies on steel poles and the big, white, washing machine? They all look to be in ideal condition so I consider this to be an ideal spot." (For what I'm not sure.)

Every day when I arrived he would be thrilled to tears to see me, although most of the time he had no idea who I was, but each night he would be just as equally shocked to realize that I had to leave him. I would read to him a lot during those days in the hospital and he seemed to enjoy it, not that he could follow the story, but the sound of my voice seemed to soothe and comfort him. One afternoon, I had been reading for a long time when he finally drifted off to sleep. Thinking to take a breather, I closed the book, but his neighbour in the next bed suddenly spoke up.

He said, "Please don't stop! I'm enjoying it."

I hadn't realized I had an audience but not wanting to disappoint him, I continued reading again.

When his son came into his room one day to visit he asked his dad how he was doing.

Edwin replied, "Well, I'm fine, but these chess men will have to go. Otherwise we'll just have to cut them all in half."

We had no idea where that came from. However, it depressed me to hear him. It was so sad to see such an elegant man reduced to mere babble and I shed many tears on his behalf. In fact, I'd cried so much already, I felt completely drained, wrung out, yet I just couldn't seem to stop.

During his stay in the hospital, Edwin began referring to his hearing aids as "fish-hooks." At least I knew what he meant! However, I probably should have removed them during the time he was there. Unfortunately, I didn't and one day his good hearing aid disappeared. I was quite upset, as it was new and very expensive, but a thorough search by the nurse, and later by myself, proved fruitless. It was gone, thrown away, no doubt, with his used Kleenex, probably carefully wrapped up in them, as was his habit those days. Unfortunately too, the garbage had already been collected and compacted so it was too late to retrieve anything—believe me, I checked!

At the end of two weeks, after the assessment of my husband had been completed, the doctor called me in to see him and I expected to be given permission to take Edwin home soon, since he seemed so much better. Thus I was totally unprepared for his pronouncement that my husband would not be coming home again but must go into a nursing home.

I was shocked!

"But I'm not ready for that!" I cried. "Edwin's not ready to go into a nursing home yet. It's too early! I can't do that!"

The doctor was sympathetic, but adamant!

"You may not be ready, my dear, but he is," he stated. "Both for your safety, and his, he must be in a nursing home. Therefore, either you find a placement for him or we will place him in the first long-term-care facility that becomes available. You have no choice in the matter other than this."

He was serious and would brook no argument.

That night sleep evaded me, as I tossed and turned, agonizing over the doctor's ultimatum and the effect it would have on poor Edwin. The following day I received a call from the social worker at the hospital, phoning to discuss Edwin's transferral to the nursing home. He mentioned that he'd had a long talk with my husband and realized his complete inability to comprehend what was happening to him, or even where he was, or what point of time he was living in at that moment. He then went on to say that he recognized the fact that whoever had been caring for him must have been having a very hard time of it. When I told him that I had been looking after him, he was amazed, frankly, that I'd managed to hold out for as long as I had. He also felt this move to a long-term-care facility was very necessary—and long overdue.

The next morning I was still reeling from shock! Until that point I had avoided checking out any nursing homes because I just couldn't bring myself to do so. In my heart of hearts, I think I felt that if I didn't do it, it wouldn't happen, it wouldn't come to this. Nevertheless, I realized now that I'd better get busy and do my homework, since I knew there were many places in which I'd never want my husband to be subjected to living, if you could even call it living! (The conditions in some of the so-called nursing homes I'd seen in the past, in my view, suggested the term "*existing*," more than "*living*," and I certainly didn't want to subject him to one of those places.) Thus, with the help of the gerontologist, I began to make a list of all the good nursing homes I'd heard about and started to check them out, conscientiously taking tours of their facilities, trying to remain objective, but still unable to picture my husband in any of them.

It was a very depressing pursuit and I grew steadily more discouraged. The greatest shock for me was in touring some of the floors dedicated to Alzheimer's patients in various stages of the disease, as I was appalled by the degree of senility among those people, and the repetitive nature of so many of their antics and actions. I convinced myself that Edwin was not like any of them and would never fit in. I still saw him as relatively normal, at least in my own mind, except of course when he'd have a bad spell, such as the other night. I think I was still in denial as to the severity of his dementia, for I still pictured him as my husband in many ways, and what he used to be, unable to face what he was becoming—or had already become. However, I dutifully made my list, citing four nursing homes in order of preference and submitting the application to the Government Placement Authorities as instructed.

Leisureworld was the name of a home in our area, and one of a chain of nursing homes in Ontario. It was a privately run facility, as opposed to government operated, and was therefore my fourth and last choice, so you can imagine my chagrin when they were the first to offer me a room—a private one—on the Alzheimer's floor. I was already shaken and miserable from having visited many other facilities, so by the time I entered the Leisureworld Nursing Home, it was with some trepidation that I rode up in the elevator with the administrator, who was taking me to see the room they had available. However, I was totally unprepared for the horrifying scene that would greet my arrival. Stepping out on to the Alzheimer's floor, my senses were so assailed by the sights and smells of the many pathetic people I saw in various stages of Alzheimer's Disease, and the noise and chaos that greeted me as I was immediately surrounded by an array of patients in various stages of dress—and undress—parading around me, that I was literally in shock. Some were walking or shuffling about, while others were in wheelchairs or nursing chairs; some whined or shouted, while others called out or came over to touch me, or to ask a question, or to seek a hug. It was appalling, utterly overwhelming, and I burst into tears!

"I can't do this," I thought!

"I can't do this to Edwin! How could he ever exist under such conditions?" I just wanted to run away, to lash out, to scream, to do anything except be there in that place!

With sympathetic understanding, the administrator calmly directed me to the available room, pointing out that we could bring some of my husband's own furniture and pictures to decorate the walls and make the place cozy and comfortable for him. She also emphasized the fact that since it was a private room he could always close the door when he wanted privacy or seclusion, and with his own things there, it could become an inviting retreat, a quiet haven from the world outside his room. Under her intuitive "handling," I finally managed to get my emotions under control and realized the potential of what she was offering. After all, he didn't have to mix with that eclectic group out in the hallway if he didn't want to do so. Then too, as I thought of some of the less-than-desirable places I'd seen, I realized that I really had no choice at this point. Anyway, I consoled myself with the thought that when one of my other choices eventually came available, I could always move him.

Thus I comforted my aching heart.

I might just explain at this point, that my first visit to the Alzheimer's ward was in the late afternoon, which was probably the worst time I could have chosen to go, since most of the patients there also suffer from some form of Sundowner's Syndrome. Throughout the years of visiting my husband in the nursing home, that continued to be the worst time of day, both for the patients and the staff. During that time also I developed a great deal of respect and admiration for the nurses and staff at the home, being impressed by their dedication and caring amidst such chaos. For most of them it was not just a job. It was much more than that, it was something they cared about deeply. They cared for the patients themselves, and I'm certain the patients and their families as well, were aware of their feelings and encouraged by them. I know I was, and I know too that I shall always hold a very special place in my heart for those dedicated workers at the Leisureworld Nursing Home.

You'll be interested to know too, that when my first choice for another nursing home did become available, I turned it down! Edwin had settled in so well at Leisureworld, and the entire staff had proven to be so wonderful and caring, I knew that I could never find a better place for him. I've discovered since, of course, that there are many wonderful nursing homes available, but for us this was definitely the best! However, there were many more hurdles to be crossed yet before coming to that conclusion, and my struggles at that juncture of the illness were just beginning, as I faced still another phase of this devastating disease.

As one doctor expressed it, "Just because the patient goes into a nursing home it doesn't mean that your troubles are over. Now you have to face a whole set of new ones!"—and he was right!

Search and Rescue

CHAPTER 14

Arriving at the nursing home the morning after Edwin had moved in, I found him walking around in the hallway, wearing only his underwear. Totally oblivious of his apparel (or lack thereof) he was out looking for me. He still didn't know my name of course, or that I was his wife, but he was looking for me nonetheless, his personal caregiver that he'd obviously become used to having around. Needless to say, he was very pleased to see me. Managing to get him properly dressed at last, I settled him into a comfortable chair in his room and began reading to him. Some time later, the nurse came into the room and announced that she wanted to give him a shower after dinner that evening.

"Why?" inquired Edwin, "Am I dirty?"

The nurse explained that it was just routine and left to do her rounds. Shortly after that Edwin went into the lavatory to use the toilet but he was in there so long I decided to check up on him. Opening the door I found him, just standing there in the middle of his washroom, stark naked! Apparently he thought his shower was to happen there and then, although there was no shower in his room, only a toilet and sink. Of course, that necessitated our having to initiate the dressing procedure all over again.

The following day the resident doctor came to visit my husband while I was there. He talked to him for quite a while, trying to test his memory, in order to gauge his level of understanding, but finally reached the same conclusion as everyone else, that he had no idea as to where he was, both in place or time. During his visit, Edwin tried to refer the doctor's attention, three separate times, to an article in the newspaper, which he seemed to feel the doctor would be interested in reading.

He kept saying, "Here Doctor, you must look at this marvellous article in the newspaper. I'm sure you would find it worthwhile reading."

However, when the doctor finally capitulated and looked at the newspaper to which Edwin was referring, he was pointing to the classified section, and, he was holding it upside down!

That one incident spoke volumes to the doctor.

For the first few months Edwin was in the nursing home, I spent hours with him every day, arriving each morning after breakfast and remaining often until nine o'clock at night when he retired. I took him to every activity they offered at Leisureworld, including a few excursions as a group to see a play, go sightseeing, shopping, or to enjoy the Christmas lights tour. He enjoyed the outings and the activities for a while, but eventually was unable to continue doing so as his condition steadily worsened. Until then however, and even long after, I tried every way possible to give him some "quality of life" to brighten up his days and bring him some happiness, no matter how fleeting.

A new doctor was coming one day, in order to do some tests on my husband and give him a physical examination, so I arrived even earlier at the home that morning in order to meet him. Later that same day I left for a dental appointment that had been scheduled several months before, following which I attended to some personal matters, such as banking and paying bills etc. On my return to the nursing home, I discovered that Edwin had tried to leave the residence, setting off all the alarms! Poor Edwin! They weren't too happy with him as you can imagine—but then again, neither was he with them. It must have been terribly frightening for him though, hearing all those alarms going off! I guess he just figured I'd been gone too long so he went looking for me. At any rate he sure wasn't too happy about it. I'd brought him a nice treat though, so that helped to mollify him somewhat. It was a chocolate bar, his favourite, so after I'd calmed him down, he munched it contentedly in his room.

Life in the nursing home was anything but boring. Besides the scheduled activities, Edwin had his own diversions, unplanned perhaps, but they certainly kept us busy nonetheless. One day his slippers disappeared, and though we spent a long time looking for them, searching high and low, they were never to be found again. Another day he lost the remote control for his television set. Apparently he'd been carrying it around in his hand the night before. This time we did find it, in someone else's room, although we had a hard time claiming it again, as that person thought it belonged to him, since it was in his room (Children, and their toys!). It could get pretty frustrating at times, trying to keep track of all his things, and of course, he'd never remember what he'd done with them. It became almost like a game for us, trying to locate all his lost articles. I'd call it *"Search and Rescue!"* He'd hide things, or leave them lying around somewhere, and I'd have to find them, with Edwin in tow. Of course we had to look everywhere, not just in his room but also anywhere on his floor, and there were lots of rooms to search in too. Many times I'd find his belongings in a room at the opposite end of the hall from his. He didn't stop with his own things either. He'd see something interesting in another patient's room and decide it should be his, so he'd take it, or perhaps he'd trade it for one of his things. Whatever the case, we'd have to play the game of "Search and Rescue" almost daily, trying to find his missing articles or perhaps attempting to find the owner of some new possession he'd acquired. Either way, it could be extremely frustrating, but it did keep us occupied. Geography was no problem for him either as he traversed the hallways many times in a day. I guess it was good exercise for him though.

When visiting, I'd often take him for a walk too, along his hall or downstairs to the basement where I'd take him to the snack store for an ice cream cone or a cappuccino, both of which he really enjoyed. In good weather I'd also take him outside for a walk down the street, while he was still capable of walking that distance, and later, when he was no longer able to go so far, in the enclosed park at the home.

On several occasions I'd arrive at the Home to find Edwin's room a disaster area. Often he would dump out all his drawers, scattering their contents throughout the room. He'd also tear the bedding off the bed, and pillows, comforters, sheets, and blankets would be thrown about in disarray, covering the chairs and the dresser but mostly on the floor. When asked what he was doing he would just say that he was looking for something, or whatever else came to mind. One day I asked him why he had made such a mess, and what he was looking for?

He declared, "Well I'm looking for boxes, of course, to ship all my files."

Obviously, he thought I should have known. I was inclined to be quite upset when those days occurred, but the nurses assured me it was normal behaviour in Alzheimer's patients. Of course I realized they must be right, but I still had a hard time dealing with it, especially as he kept on losing his belongings, which sure didn't help. Some of his things I ended up having to take home with me, as he just couldn't look after them any more. One such item was his wedding ring, which he'd lost a total of three times, but the nurses had managed to find it again on all three occasions, amazingly enough. After the third time, however, the nurse handed it to me and requested that I take it home, as they didn't want to be responsible for it any more. I can't say I blamed them either!

One day I was more upset than usual on finding his room a mess once again and I burst into tears, so later on, when it was time for her break, the head nurse, Janet, came in for a visit. We had a long chat, which was most helpful, and I shall always be grateful for this lovely, young woman taking the time to help me through yet another hurdle in my journey with Alzheimer's.

The essence of her advice to me was that I should come to the home every day *expecting the worst*. Then, if I found things in a state of disaster, it was only to be expected, so I couldn't be disappointed. However, if things were okay when I arrived—or even better—then it would be a pleasant surprise, as I hadn't expected it. Now that may sound like negative thinking, and perhaps it was in a sense, but the outcome of such reasoning was positive, and that's what counted, so I had to learn to adjust my own perspective. In reality I had always enjoyed a positive, upbeat personality, trusting people and thinking the best of them, until proven otherwise of course. In fact, I was even gullible and naïve in some ways. Therefore, such a convoluted way of thinking was totally opposite to my natural inclinations, but nonetheless, I realized I'd better adjust, if I wanted to survive. It did help too—a lot!

One other truth that Janet tried to emphasize for me, and perhaps the hardest to accept, was the need to face the reality of the fact that *things were only going to get worse* from that point on—not better—and I needed to be prepared. It was difficult to hear my worst fears confirmed, put into words as it were, and expressed as a reality, not just a concept. Even then I found it hard to accept, but I knew she was right.

With Alzheimer's one can only go forward—never backwards. The past has gone, never to be restored, and the only direction is ahead.

The following day Edwin's watch was missing but fortunately, I found it under his bed. Sometimes it would be his teeth, another time his glasses, or his hearing aid, or his watch. Then too, it might be all his socks that were missing, or all his handkerchiefs, or whatever else he decided to dump on any given day. I never bought as many socks or handkerchiefs in my life as I did during those years with Edwin in the nursing home. I sure don't know where all his things disappeared to, even to this day, but they did. Everything was labelled as well, but it made no difference. All his possessions had his name and room number on them, no matter how small, but they could still disappear, often without a trace! (And you think your washing machine swallows socks!)

Eventually the nurses gave me all of Edwin's special belongings to take home (at least what was left of them), before everything disappeared. This included his wedding ring, which he'd lost several times as mentioned earlier, and his latest watch, as well as the television remote and anything else that wasn't fastened to the wall or out of reach. In one of his destructive moods he even broke the aerial off the television set, and another time he tore the plug out of the wall, leaving the wires bare and the plug still in the receptacle. Of course the TV wouldn't work after that but it didn't seem to bother him.

One day the nurse tried to explain to me why my husband always had such a load of laundry each week. Apparently he had taken to undressing several times a day, and since the nurses never knew which of his clothes were clean or dirty, they'd just start over, dressing him again in something fresh from his cupboard. Actually, at one point I had a lock installed on his closet, so that became one less place to get trashed.

Some days, still, I would find the entire situation very trying and frustrating. However, there was one major difference that helped me during those days with Edwin in the nursing home. Now that he was in a long-term facility, being cared for 24 hours a day, I could leave when I needed to, or when things got too much for me, and go for a walk outside, or for a meal, or just a cup of coffee. Then I would return in a better frame of mind, more able to cope with the situation. That was a tremendous difference from being with him at home by myself, day and night, and having no chance of retreat; no opportunity to recoup my sanity, and for that I was grateful.

Soon after his entering the nursing home I discovered a new addition to my husband's wardrobe, incontinent underwear. I was shocked to discover this new development, but he didn't appear to mind at all. He seemed to accept the situation as normal and not in the least demeaning or humiliating. In fact, he even referred to himself as dressing like Gandhi, and was quite proud of the fact. (That memory stemmed from his years in India, no doubt.) I guess it did make sense. At least it relieved the workload for the nurses, creating less laundry, and probably taking some of the pressure off Edwin as well. However, I would never have dared to introduce such a measure for fear of humiliating him or diminishing his self-esteem. Maybe I shouldn't have been so protective of his feelings all that time; who knows? Anyway, his calm acceptance of all those changes just amazed me.

During his first few weeks in the Home, Edwin was permitted to take his meals in the main dining room downstairs. However, in time that arrangement turned out to be a disaster. Poor Edwin never knew where to go, from one mealtime to the next, so someone always had to escort him to the dining room if I wasn't there, and often he'd get lost trying to find his way back home after the meal, especially if someone didn't get to him soon enough, because when he was ready to leave there was no stopping him.

On speaking about the experience, Edwin commented, "The *exiting* seems very *exciting* at the time, but when you get there and discover you're entirely on your own, it's frightening!"

Eventually they had to stop that practice, after he got lost a few times too many, and transferred his meals to the dining room on his own floor.

Before that time came though, on arriving at the home shortly after 8:00 a.m. one morning, I was surprised in not finding Edwin in the dining room downstairs. Walking up to his floor, I located him in his own dining room, and the reason he had not been permitted to go downstairs as usual was patently obvious. He certainly wouldn't have met the dress code, not that there was one actually. However, that morning his attire was bizarre and would have been unthinkable downstairs. Apparently when the nurse went into his room to dress him that day, she had found him already dressed, at least by his own declaration, and ready to go for breakfast. Not wanting to argue with him, especially so early in the morning, she allowed him to remain as he was, but directed him to the dining room on his own floor instead of the other one. His costume that morning consisted of blue pyjama pants and a striped pyjama shirt, with an undershirt on top and a beige sweater vest buttoned over that. Another undershirt was wrapped around his shoulders like a shawl, and topping off this "ensemble" was a long, brown knee sock, wound around his neck like a scarf. A handkerchief, so-called, consisting of long legged under shorts the colour of mustard, was stuck into his shirt pocket and used occasionally to wipe his nose. The nurses were rather embarrassed at my having found him in that state of dress but I hastened to assure them of my understanding.

"After all," I reminded them, "don't forget I used to live with him!

One day when I was visiting Edwin, it became apparent that he thought he was being kept in his room as a punishment for having misbehaved.

He said to me, tears in his eyes, "When I was a child my mother used to ask me if I'd learned my lesson yet. Well, I hadn't then, but I have now."

"Oh, love, you are not being punished!" I said, hastening to assure him, while tears filled my eyes as well. "That's not why you're here!"

"Yes it is," he cried, plaintively, "I know I've been a bad boy, but I've learned my lesson. I'll be good now! You'll see!"

He was so pathetic and sounded so forlorn, it broke my heart, making me weep. After that I just stood there hugging him for a long time, until we both stopped crying, but I never forgot his words that day, and I doubt I ever will. Even now it brings tears to my eyes, just thinking about it—remembering the pathos of the moment.

When I took Edwin for his last appointment with the psychiatrist, a follow-up to his hospital stay and subsequent move to the nursing home, the doctor asked him where he was living now.

Edwin replied, "I can't remember the name of the hotel," looking at me to supply the answer, as always.

The doctor winked at me and said, "Well maybe your wife can tell us the name of the hotel."

It would appear that he still had no idea that he was living in a nursing home, and I certainly didn't want to be the one to abuse him of his fantasies, nor did the doctor obviously, so we let it go. Whatever worked for him!

It was such a beautiful day outside, so after the doctor's appointment I took him for an ice cream cone, which he loved. I ended up wearing most of his cone myself, but he enjoyed it immensely, so it was worth it. I didn't mind at all. I was just glad to see him looking so happy and content. It was quite a contrast to his usual demeanour.

One Sunday we drove over to his son's house for dinner with the family. Edwin was on his best behaviour, which pleased me no end, but I think the whole experience was a real eye-opener for the others.

At one point Edwin asked me, "Do I need to go to the bathroom?"

I replied, "I really don't know, but I'd be glad to take you if you want to try."

He did!

All considered, it was a good visit and he ate a healthy amount, but I think the occasion was very hard on his son especially, seeing his father in such a deteriorated condition. The entire evening was rather strained and I'm sure he was relieved when we left—I know Edwin was too.

Once back at the Home, I had an extremely hard time getting away. Poor Edwin was totally confused and agitated and I finally had to get the head nurse to remain with him in his room, while I escaped. She mentioned to me the next day that his behaviour in reaction to the preceding evening was actually quite normal with Alzheimer's patients, and that I should not be overly concerned. She explained that going out, especially to another home for a period of time, usually upsets them quite severely, as it breaks their schedule, which they've already become used to, so she suggested quite strongly that it was not advisable to attempt it too often. I had to agree with her after that experience. Short walks or jaunts were fine, but prolonged visits away from the Home were just too difficult for him to sustain at that stage, and I realized we needed to avoid them in the future if at all possible.

Some days on my visits to Edwin he would be extremely talkative, going on non-stop about anything and everything. Unfortunately, most of it rarely made any sense. Other days however, he'd just sit and stare into space, his face muscles hanging slack, and the drool dribbling down his chin and chest. Then I would know that he was far away from me—somewhere I couldn't reach. Sadly, as the disease progressed, those days occurred more frequently, until they just took over and he became totally lost to me and everyone else.

He had no idea who I was at all any more and he could never remember my name. The nurses would keep telling him that his wife was coming but he wouldn't believe them. Then when I'd arrive he would always look surprised—and pleased—but still he'd think I was just a figment of his imagination. One day one of the patients referred to me as Edwin's *friend*.

He corrected her immediately, saying, "She's not my friend, she's an employee of this place!"

I really thought he was going to say *my wife*, and I was disappointed. (There I was, getting my hopes up again. I just couldn't seem to learn!)

Another time one of the workers mentioned his wife to Edwin, knowing that I came to visit every day, but he told her that his wife had been dead for months. (Not years, just months.) I have no idea why he thought I was dead, but obviously he did.

Thus the days moved on, one after the other, the days turning into weeks, the weeks turning into months, and the months, years. It was always difficult to say goodbye to Edwin each evening as I left for home. He would try to follow me down the hall, or watch me through the tiny window of the stairwell, looking pathetic and crestfallen, for even though he didn't know who I was, he knew I was someone who cared, and he hated to see me go.

It used to tear at my heartstrings, taking my leave, and I tried to devise less traumatic ways of accomplishing it. Instead of saying goodbye, I learned to say "I'll see you later," suggesting to him that I'd be back that same day. If I said "tomorrow" he'd get upset, but "later" (that same day) seemed better, and he didn't know one day from another anyway. As well, I learned to coincide my departures with his meal times, whenever possible, seating him in the dining room at the table, telling him his dinner was coming and that I'd see him later. That ploy worked best of all, so that's the one we finally adopted. With his thoughts concentrated on food, he'd forget that I wasn't there.

As it was, he never knew that I'd been there from one day to the next, or even one hour to the next, and when I'd return on the same day it would be as though it was my first visit. However, he was always very glad to see me and greeted me anew, no matter how many times I'd return in one day.

The Lost Foot

Time continued to pass, slowly and inexorably moving forward, even as the disease took its course, until the day came when I realized, to my surprise, that Edwin had been in the nursing home for eight months already. Frankly, I was amazed! I didn't know where that time had gone. It just went, as did the months and years that followed, one day after the next. During the past eight months, Edwin had settled in surprisingly well. He no longer needed special medication, except for nights, and for the most part was quite content. He still had his times of course, and I never knew what to expect from day to day, but I continued to drop by for a few hours every day to visit with him, and he always had a few surprises up his sleeve, to keep me on my toes, as it were.

During those long months, I learned to exercise a lot of patience but still had days when I found it difficult to accept some of his behaviour. At least now, though, I could leave and go for a walk or something, if I needed to get away, returning shortly but somewhat refreshed and more able to cope. Of course, nothing in life is all black and white and dealing with dementia was no different. There were also moments of laughter along the way, as some of his antics were pretty funny at best and even if laughter was out of the question, there were times I had to smile, however sadly. The tears were always very close at hand and sometimes intermingled with the laughter so that I would find myself at a loss, wondering whether to laugh or cry, a situation that often plagued me during those long, dark days and even afterwards for some time. However, I do maintain that in many cases it was my sense of humour that kept me going. Without it I never could have survived. In some situations one can *only* laugh or cry so how much better it is to laugh, if you can!

I walked into his room one day, giving him my usual, bright, cheery greeting. No recognition of course, he never recognized me anymore by then, but his rejoinder was immediate and stated almost indignantly.

"I'm short a foot!"

"What do you mean?" I asked, puzzled.

"I've lost a foot!"

Glancing at his feet (a natural response), and noting they were both there, (not that I expected otherwise) I replied somewhat inanely, "Oh really?" not knowing what else to say.

"Yes," he reiterated, "I've lost a foot! The shoe's gone too!"

"But they're both there," I said, "I can see them."

"No they're not!" he insisted.

Having absolutely no idea what he was talking about, my mind started to consider all the possibilities. I sat him down and removed his shoes and socks, putting both his feet up on a stool. Thinking, perhaps, that one of his feet had gone to sleep, I gently massaged them for a while before putting his shoes back on. I still have no idea what his problem was, but he enjoyed the massage—and the attention—so was quite content after that. Poor Edwin just couldn't seem to express himself anymore. He still had lots of words but just didn't know how to use them. I felt so maternal towards him. He was no longer my husband, hadn't been for some time in fact, as he seemed more like an infant to me, but I loved him very much as I would my child.

Sometime after that particular episode I learned that people with Alzheimer's, in their inability to express their thoughts lucidly, will often use words that are opposite to those intended. That certainly rang true for me, as Edwin used to tell people how I'd fixed the kitchen ceiling at home some time ago, when in actuality I'd fixed the bathroom floor. Also he'd speak of his hand when referring to his foot. One time he was desperately searching for his glasses. When I found them and gave them to him he was most upset at me, insisting that they weren't what he wanted.

"I want the long thin ones," he insisted, finally satisfied when I handed him his pen.

In looking back, I realize that I had absolutely no inkling of what he was referring to, the day he *lost his foot*. However, whatever it was he was trying to express, he was effectively diverted from it becoming an issue when he enjoyed his foot massage, and that in itself was a blessing. In fact, anything that prevented a subject from becoming an issue could be a blessing, as issues had a habit of escalating out of hand and blowing up in your face. Believe me, I know! That was definitely something to be avoided—at any cost!

One day when I came for my regular visit, both the doctor and the head nurse greeted me in my husband's room. Whenever there was an incident of any kind it was common practice for the doctor to examine the patient and determine the extent of injury—if any— even though in most cases there was no evident trauma. Of course, it was more in the nature of preventative medicine, as people at that stage of Alzheimer's don't seem to feel pain as they used to, and some problems could go unnoticed before becoming major concerns. In fact, the absence of pain was often what enabled them to accomplish great feats of strength, such as when Edwin threw the nurse against the wall even though she was twice his size. When they don't feel pain, they don't know their limitations either, and can harm themselves simply by overextending or overtaxing their abilities. At any rate, they always made sure, by checking out anyone involved in an incident or a fall, no matter how seemingly minor it might have been.

On that particular day, the nurse began to relate the current episode to me. It seems that one of the other patients on Edwin's floor, a tiny woman with a penchant for constantly walking—more like marching really—had an altercation with one of the nurses and slapped the beleaguered nurse across the face. Bristling with anger, she had then proceeded to stomp up the hallway until accosting my husband, he being the first person she encountered after the nurse. Still in an aggressive frame of mind, and in no mood to brook interference, she mustered all the force her diminutive stature would allow and slapped Edwin across the face too. Poor Edwin, totally taken aback, responded by reciprocating the attack and slapping her across the face as well.

"It was no small slap," said the nurse. "She really gave it to him and Edwin gave it right back! In fact," she said, "He didn't just slap her. He really let her have it!"

At that point Edwin's face lit up and he exclaimed proudly, "I didn't even know I *had* it!"

Needless to say, we doubled up laughing, and Edwin laughed along with us. He didn't realize, of course, that he'd actually made a joke but he enjoyed sharing in our laughter.

Actually, it is quite a common occurrence for someone with Alzheimer's to pick up on one sentence of a conversation and respond—often quite intelligently in fact—to that one sentence. In most cases the comment is completely out of context with the subject being discussed, as it was in that case, since they are unable to follow a conversation but do hear isolated phrases. Often too, their response is several subjects behind that particular point in the conversation, so it can throw others off course, especially if they've already gone on to other topics. When my husband would do that, he'd have no idea that he was "out of context" or going backwards in the discussion. He just wanted to be part of it, to belong as it were. Realizing his motivation, we could cater to him, causing him to become inordinately pleased by a simple, polite response such as "Really!" or, "Is that so?" or, "That's very interesting!" or, "Well, aren't you clever to realize that!" and so on, as the occasion allowed. On the other hand, we could make him feel frustrated or confused by questioning his response, causing him to head off down a blind alley conversationally, getting flustered and coming to an abrupt stop. Any conversation was over his head by that time, but he still liked to feel that he was participating, as long as he wasn't put on the spot by having his response questioned. He simply was not able to follow through with any further comment, and would totally lose the trend of his thoughts, such as they were.

Conversely, another interesting quality of Alzheimer's patients at times, is their amazing ability to hang on to a specific thought, sometimes tenuously, bringing it up over and over again, and Edwin was no exception in that regard. It could apply to a question that he'd ask repeatedly, even though I'd already answered it dozens of times, or it could be something he wanted to do which was totally impossible, such as *going home*. Then again, it could involve a conversation which may have progressed ten minutes or more beyond a certain subject, when he'd suddenly make a comment pertaining to that previous object of discussion. That could also prove somewhat disconcerting for those conversing, as their mindset had already passed on to a new subject, while he would still be ruminating on what was discussed previously (usually limited to one sentence only though, and not the entire conversation). Again, a simple, conventional response to his comment would put his mind at ease and please him no end, as he'd feel he had contributed his bit to the conversation. The fact that it was totally irrelevant or out of context had no bearing on his pleasure whatever, as long as it wasn't pointed out to him, of course.

In that same vein, Edwin would often come out with comments totally unrelated to the present day and age. Since the short-term memory is the first to go in Alzheimer's patients, they usually live in the past, which fact is reflected by much of their conversation. For instance, if Edwin talked about his mother, it was always in the present. Sometimes he'd be convinced she was still alive. Rather than trying to argue the point, which was impossible anyway, since his mind was already made up, I'd try to change the subject by asking him to tell me about his mother.

"What was she like?"

"What was your home like?"

"Tell me about your mother."

As he would answer each question to the best of his ability, he'd slowly become diverted from whatever else he'd introduced into the conversation. Of course, I'd only ask one question at a time, rather than asking them all at once, since, as I mentioned before, he was unable to handle multiple questions.

Before I learned that lesson for myself, I used to ask my husband questions such as, "Would you like some coffee, or tea, or juice?"

He'd simply reply, "Yes, please."

Then I'd have to start all over again, asking him one thing at a time. I did learn, eventually, but it took time and it seemed to me that I always learned everything the hard way.

Nothing's ever easy! Life itself isn't easy, but I learned to be thankful for the good days, even as I got used to the bad ones. I also learned to heed the admonition of the head nurse, Janet, and always to expect the worst! That way the good days were a gift, and the bad days weren't so disappointing as they were only to be expected. As I said before, life has no guarantees and you learn to accept the good with the bad. It's a hard lesson to learn but it's the only way to salvage your sanity and peace of mind, and goodness knows we all need as much of that as we can get.

Those days too, I was busy packing, preparing for the move from our house to the condo we'd bought, the new home that Edwin would never get to live in. Instead of being a happy occasion, it loomed more as a sad one, an unhappy ending to a chapter of our lives together. However, it only hurt to look backwards, so I pressed on, trying to look forward and remain positive, at least when I was with my husband. It was important for me to keep his spirits up and I tried my best to be happy and cheerful in his company, as pleasant and positive as I could, but believe me, it wasn't always easy—or possible. The tears were never far away from the surface those days, although I tried to reserve that luxury for the privacy of my own home and many were the days I wept copious tears while driving my car, returning home from a visit with Edwin. At times I could hardly see the road through my tears and some days I'd have to pull over to the side of the highway until I could get my emotions under control.

During the busy task of packing (I hate moving at the best of times, especially on my own), I got into the habit of going to the nursing home in the evening, instead of having to change clothes twice in the middle of the day. One evening on my arrival, I found his room uncomfortably cool, so I called Andrew, the maintenance man and a very nice chap, to come and fix the heater, which he did. Afterwards I asked Edwin to feel the radiator to see if it was working.

He walked over to the television set, felt it, and declared, "Yes, it's warm."

Again, I had to smile!

Arriving at the nursing home one morning, I found Edwin with Luna, a lovely girl from Activation, getting ready to go downstairs for games so I went along with them to accompany my husband during the program. The Activation Department in a nursing home is the one concerned with keeping the patients busy and active, and Luna, the girl directly responsible for Edwin's floor, was very good at her chosen career. Along with Annie and Andrew, the head of the department, and all the other workers and volunteers, they did a wonderful job working with the patients and were very good to Edwin and me. I really appreciated what they were doing and their dedication to the task, which was not easy at the best of times. I know; I was there! That day, Luna confided in me that she was becoming very discouraged with Edwin's lack of progress. He used to try to please her and she enjoyed working with him, but now his lack of response was discouraging to say the least. Then, adding to this, one day he really scared her, grabbing at her with a wild expression in his eyes. She was encouraged to hear that I had also noticed a change in him and that it was not just her that was having a problem, but she was saddened too, realizing that his regression into the disease was becoming more apparent.

That morning they served lovely muffins after the program and I fed Edwin his, giving him one morsel at a time. He kept growling at me and snatching at each piece with his teeth. Not wanting to encourage this behaviour, I tried to get him to eat the muffin by himself, but ended up having to put each individual piece into his hand, directing him then to put it into his own mouth. It was a slow and laborious task and just as I was beginning to wonder if it was worth the effort, dear Annie came over to say that they were glad to see I was making Edwin do things for himself. She told me then that although it's not possible to teach an Alzheimer's patient anything new, it is important to reaffirm what they do know. That was certainly encouraging to me and I continued to persevere until the muffin was finished.

When I gave Edwin a new watch for his birthday he was very pleased. He had lost his previous one—in fact he'd lost several already including a couple his son had given to him—but he loved having a watch on his wrist. Of course, I no longer invested in expensive ones, just ten dollar ones, and the digital kind, since he had not been able to read a regular clock face for a long time by then. At any rate he was extremely happy with his new watch and as I left him that day he was beaming with pleasure. However, the next day when I came to visit, he complained that his new watch was not working.

"This watch is no good!" he said. "It doesn't work."

I looked at it and found it to be keeping perfect time so I told him so, showing him the correct time.

"Well," he said, "I guess there are a few good minutes left in this one after all!"

I had to laugh. He had such a unique way of expressing himself at times.

Edwin found a new friend in the nursing home, a sweet man named Alex, who called himself Alexander the Great. He was really a cute little man with large blue eyes and a beatific smile. Obviously a cat lover in his day, he was always carrying around a few stuffed animals—cats of course—whenever I saw him. One day I found him sitting beside Edwin on the chairs in the hall, as usual, his arms filled with stuffed kittens.

Alex looked up at me and said, "You look so nice with your fur coat, and your nice earrings—and your nice teeth!"

I almost choked on that last bit!

He then turned to Edwin and asked, "Do you like cat food?"

"I can't remember." was Edwin's thoughtful reply.

The interaction between patients could be quite amusing at times and usually gave me a good chuckle.

One day Edwin introduced me to one of the workers. She and I then started talking until Edwin interrupted.

"You two act as though you know one another!" he remarked.

"We do know each other," we both replied.

Quite upset, Edwin then complained, "Can't I introduce you to anyone?"

Another time, on escorting Edwin to the dining room for dinner, I seated him at a table with three women, which Edwin always enjoyed.

One of the women, on realizing a man was seated at her table, declared, "We can't have a man at our table! We're all going to get pregnant!"

Edwin's regular visit to the dentist came around again, and I picked him up to drive him to his appointment. Going to the dentist was really quite a trek for both of us as his office was at the top of a flight of long, steep stairs. Getting up the stairs was bad enough, but going down them afterwards was extremely difficult, to say the least. The dentist would always send one of his girls to help us accomplish the feat, but Edwin would need instructions for each, individual step, forgetting after each one what he was supposed to do next, and it would be a long and precarious ordeal. I always breathed a sigh of relief when we reached the bottom and I'm sure the dentist's assistant did as well.

Afterwards we went out for lunch and then over to Alma's for coffee, all of which Edwin enjoyed immensely. It was definitely one of his better days and a delightful outing.

Even so, as we were getting ready to leave Alma's place she commented to me, "I don't know how you do it!"

On leaving, I remarked on the weather, just musing out loud really, wondering if it was still raining or if there'd been any let-up, since it hadn't been a good day at all, in that regard.

Edwin replied immediately, "I can't think of any valid reason why there should be, unless it's pure clumsiness on their part."

Where that came from, I've no idea, but Alma and I both enjoyed a good laugh!

On another occasion, when I admonished Edwin not to try tying his own shoelaces anymore, after I'd spent hours untying all the knots in them, he was quick to defend himself.

"It was done by the police!" he avowed.

Incredulous, I asked "Why would the police want to tie knots in your laces?"

"Because," he replied, "They were all chivvying about by themselves."

I'm sure it made perfect sense to him!

When he asked one day about the "climate" outside, I told him it was nice and sunny, but cold.

He then said, "No, I mean *depositations*! (His word, not mine.)

I just told him, "There is no snow and no rain," which seemed to satisfy him.

While attending a birthday party in the Home, where they did a lot of off-key singing, Edwin's comment reflected his photographic background.

"I wonder how they'd sound if they were *in focus*?" he said.

One day he asked me, "What about those *boxes* stacked in the corner of the room? What are they for?"

"Those aren't boxes," I tried to explain, "they're your shelves."

"Well, they were packing boxes before they were stacked as shelves then," was his indignant reply.

On being asked a question about one of his friends one day, Edwin replied, "Oh I don't know these things.

You have to sit and wallow in them for days, unless you have a five or six thousand dollar watch."

I should have known better than to ask!

When his son had a new baby boy, I shared the good news with Edwin, letting him know he had another grandchild.

I finished by saying, "Well, what do you think of that?"

He replied, "Well, what I do think is that someone drank my drink!"

He just had no concept of anything anymore. He was really out of it!

The head nurse on evenings at the Home was a very nice young man named Mike. He walked into Edwin's room one evening as usual, greeting him warmly.

"Hi Edwin, how's it going?"

"Fine, thank you," he replied.

However, after Mike left, Edwin turned to me and said, "How in hell did he know my name was Edwin?"

They say that people with Alzheimer's disease get to meet *new people* every day. I guess they're right!

One morning when I opened up Edwin's curtains to let the lovely sunshine into his room, he stared out of the window for a long, long time.

Finally I was prompted to enquire, "What are you looking at?"

"I'm just curious to see what a French onion looks like." was his reply.

I didn't ask!

Later he told me he'd started the day with a big fight. Inquiring as to why there was a big fight, I was given this answer:

"The boy came in sodden wet!"

He was probably remembering an incident that happened a long time ago, possibly with his son as the boy, although after I'd had my hair cut short he also used to refer to me as the boy, so who knows?

After all those months in the nursing home he still had to ask each time where the bathroom was located, although he had long ago reverted to using the word "lavatory" instead of toilet, and I would direct him as usual to the one in his room. One day, however, he was in there so long I decided it would be prudent to check up on him. Unfortunately, I should have gone sooner! I found him busy playing with his stool, carefully wrapping it up in toilet paper, like a treasured possession. I suggested, to his dismay, that he might want to dispose of the "package" in the toilet, which he finally did, though begrudgingly.

The entire incident totally grossed me out! I'd found those "packages" before, lying about his room, or in his dresser drawers, but until then I'd convinced myself that it had to be someone else doing it. Not him! Not my Edwin! It was unthinkable, but after that I had to face the ugly truth.

There were other times, later on, that I would find, not only a "package" in the drawer, but his feces smeared all over the walls and on his bed-side table as well. In fact, even further down the road, they had to dispose of the nice wastebasket I'd placed in his room. Apparently it wouldn't come clean after he'd used it for a "job" one day, instead of the toilet.

Sometimes I'd really have to fight my stomach over those gross occurrences. How I admired the nurses for their stamina! I don't know how they did it, day after day, but they did. Also, I was grateful that I could call the housekeeping department to clean things up for him. At times like that I was very thankful that he was in a nursing home and not still at home with only me to look after him.

Another day Edwin was seriously contemplating his buttons when I arrived. He had two left over and couldn't make them "stick."

He said, "They need juice on them to make them stick. Otherwise a sheet of rain will come and wash it away."

After listening to this strange explanation for a while, I finally showed him how to put the two remaining buttons through the buttonholes. He was quite impressed with my expertise!

Every day it was something else! Sometimes his comments were not particularly memorable, or they were just such nonsense that I couldn't follow what he said, much less remember. However, there were days that stood out in my memory and I recorded them verbatim.

One such day he said, "You know what they've done? They've taken out all the fresh fish and put in the other stuff instead!"

Another time he commented, "I can see which way business is going to take us right now!"

"Which way?" I asked.

"Firstly," he replied, "The way we want to go, and secondly, the way we will go."

Makes perfect sense—doesn't it?

When I asked him how he was doing one day, he made the following reply:

"No, the rain isn't doing anything. Everything else is doing everything!"

Another day he was really impressed with the Velcro closures on his shoes. I'd bought the shoes for him back in Florida, so he'd had them for well over a year, but he couldn't grasp the fact that they were still the same pair. He thought they were new.

A favourite expression of his was always, "And thereby hangs a tale!"

I was encouraged to hear him using it again one day, until he went on to say, "Yes, it's hanging on the other side of the door. That's where I put it."

Sometimes Edwin would be convinced that he was not allowed to use any of the lavatories (His word, not mine). Then he'd tell me that he'd like to find a men's room, but his "lavatory" wasn't there any more. Of course he still had one in his own room, but there was no use arguing with him when he'd already made up his mind so I would just wait a while.

Then I'd bring up the subject again by asking, "Would you like to go to the bathroom now?"

He'd usually answer, "Yes, please."

Then he'd allow me to take him to his own washroom, with no more argument.

Of course the key was in waiting, knowing that in time he would forget his obsession—until the next time, of course!

Most of the time, I could neither figure out where he was coming from, nor where he was going, in regard to his conversations, if you could even dignify his use of words by describing them as such. However, the humour in his comments was undeniably evident, and patently obvious, providing a perfect foil for the backdrop of pain and anguish. Sometimes I had to laugh, in spite of myself, in spite of my tears, but the laughter was good for my soul—and my sanity!

He may have lost a foot that day, but I gained a lot more. I learned to laugh at his antics, to laugh at myself, and to see the humour through my veil of tears—and I learned to survive!

Too Many Hats

Every time I visited the nursing home I'd go as a different person, at least as far as Edwin was concerned. One day I'd be a *nurse*, another day a *doctor*, or a *worker* in the Home, or even the *director* of the Home. Sometimes I'd be the *manager* of the "hotel" Edwin was living in, or just the *cook*. Once he asked me if I was *Sally Ann*, an affectionate nickname widely used for Salvation Army personnel, an organization which helps a lot of needy people. Another time I arrived directly from Church, wearing a long, white knitted skirt and sweater and he asked me if I'd just been married that day. In fact, the only occupation missing was his *wife*. He never mistook me for his wife, the one avocation that truly belonged to me. Every day I wore a *different hat* for Edwin; too many hats for me, and certainly too many for Edwin to cope with—it's no wonder he was confused! So was I! I never knew who I was going to be, from one day to the next. All I did know was that I loved him, whatever he had become, and wherever he was hiding inside that tangled brain of his, and I wanted to help him in any way I could. It wasn't always easy though. In fact, it was extremely difficult, to say the least, but I had the satisfaction of seeing him smile—if only briefly from time to time—and providing him some *quality* of life, if not *quantity*. Maybe his enjoyment was only for a moment—short-lived at best—but that was still better than none at all, and as long as I had life, I intended to dedicate that life to helping him live his to the fullest, enjoying the time he had left to the best degree possible under the circumstances. That was the hat I wanted to wear—in fact, needed to wear—in order to help him, in order to fulfill my vow.

As mentioned earlier, the various programs offered to the patients in the nursing home were conducted by the Activation Department, and they did a marvellous job of providing many opportunities for the patients to enjoy a variety of activities, requiring varying degrees of participation. As much as possible we attempted to avail ourselves of every activity feasible, partaking in as many of those occasions as time and ability would allow, and I would escort my husband to the activity room myself whenever I could.

One such endeavour was the game of bingo, which most of the patients seemed to enjoy, despite their inability, in many cases, to keep up with the caller. I would sit at a table with Edwin and three other patients, helping each one to place their bingo chips on the numbers called. *Another hat—the Bingo Lady*! If a card at our table proved to be a winner, I would also have to encourage the winning player to yell "Bingo!" at the appropriate time, at which point the winner would usually giggle in his (or her) excitement, never quite sure what to make of the situation.

Eventually, however, we had to give up on that particular pursuit, after Edwin decided the plastic bingo-chips must be cookies, or something equally edible, and started eating them—or trying to at least. Once he'd get one in his mouth, he'd refuse to spit it out or let me have it, and quite a scuffle would ensue. I'd actually have to fight with him to remove it, my fingers in his mouth, and he equally determined not to let it go. Needless to say, I was afraid he might swallow one of the chips some time—or even choke—if I didn't get it out on time, while he was similarly intent on swallowing it if he could. It made for quite a show, as the other patients cheered us on, but it proved too much for my shattered nerves, so our Bingo playing days came to an ignominious end! I'm still not sure just who the patients were rooting for in the scuffle, but then again, I'm not sure I really want to know! Suffice it to say we put the afternoons of participating in Bingo games behind us, for good. In fact, even to this day I cringe whenever I hear the game mentioned.

One day I came to the nursing home to find my husband in a terrible mood. The nurses warned me on my arrival that he didn't want to be bothered with anyone that day and he refused to let a soul near him. That explained why I found him in the condition he was in: unshaven and unkempt, still in his pyjamas, with his clothing inside out on top of them. Actually he looked quite a sight to behold, with his pant pockets hanging outside and all the bare seams showing. He also had a difficult time trying to express his thoughts that day as well, for nothing he said made any sense at all.

The following day he was in a much better frame of mind. Speaking of frames, that day also, he suddenly noticed all his pictures on the wall, as if for the first time! They'd been there for a long time already, as I'd hung them up the day before he arrived, when he moved over from the hospital his first day. At any rate, he seemed very surprised to see them and wanted to know how they were "hanged up" all of a sudden. Well, I was just glad he liked them anyway so I didn't worry about how or when they got there. That day too, he allowed me to shave him and get him dressed, which was a relief for everyone, since he hadn't per-mitted any of the nurses near him for three days. However, that day he was also demanding to be given a "bottle of scotch" and was quite upset that no one accommodated him or complied with his request. I guess we couldn't win them all!

The first Sunday in May, Leisureworld hosts all the patients and their families and friends to a wonderful Annual Spring Tea. It was always a lovely occasion and they really set it up beautifully, going out of their way to make it a delightful yearly affair to which I always enjoyed bringing Edwin, and his son when he was able to be present. A gorgeous buffet would be set up along one wall, complete with finger foods, some hot items, and sweets, along with punch, and coffee or tea. They also supplied excellent musical entertainment and, on the whole, created a tasteful, elegant atmosphere for all who attended. It was certainly one of the highlights of the year and an occasion I looked forward to as well, along with everyone I'm sure. I also enjoyed the opportunity afforded by the tea party of visiting with some of the other patient's relatives that I'd come to know through the years at the Home. It was always an enjoyable afternoon and a credit to the staff and management of the Leisureworld Nursing Home, and I'm sure everyone was appreciative of their efforts. I know I certainly was grateful.

Each year though, I would be amazed at the quantity of sweets Edwin was able to ingest at the tea party. He would patently avoid all the things I enjoyed, such as shrimp, chicken bits, devilled eggs, veggies and dip, and would head straight for the sweet tray. Of course, after his first year I had to fetch his food for him, but even so, he would only eat the sweets I brought to the table, nothing else. He loved chocolate most of all and would ask for "anything chocolatey." He'd devour any of the sweets I brought him, but the chocolate would inevitably go first. In fact, he'd ignore everything else, so eventually I learned to serve him only the sweets. I'd load a plate for him with all his favourites and just let him go to it. What difference did it make anyway? Nothing could hurt him by then, so I just let him indulge himself, as he noisily gobbled up the treats, "oohing" and "aahing" with every mouthful. Actually, it did my heart good to see him enjoying himself so much. I don't believe he was ever sick afterwards either—at least not that anyone ever reported to me. I'm sure if I had eaten all that chocolate I would have been very sick, but not Edwin!

In actuality, the entire scenario was particularly noteworthy, in my estimation—at least to me—because this was the same man who hardly ever ate desserts or sweets in his life. Only when we were out visiting would he indulge in a dessert, and then only to be polite, as he much preferred meat and potatoes, or even sandwiches, to sweets. However, I did notice that other Alzheimer's patients also indulged equally in the dessert trays, especially those who were able to serve themselves. They would all head straight for the sweets, ignoring everything else on the long buffet table. Perhaps this penchant for sugar is significant among Alzheimer's patients, or maybe it's just endemic to their return to the child in them—the child they'd become. Whatever the reason, I enjoyed watching them delighting in the treats, which made them happy—for that moment in time at least.

One morning I found Edwin sitting in the lounge area when I arrived, his trousers pushed up to his knees, and his socks pulled on over his shoes.

"I see you had some trouble putting on your socks today," I commented.

"There seems to be some trouble with them," he conceded. "They don't work!"

I took him back to his room and removed his socks and shoes, putting the socks back on his feet first, and then his shoes. He was quite impressed with my ability in *fixing them*! He honestly did not know why his socks wouldn't fit properly before.

Noticing his nice, clean hair after that, I commented on it.

"Well, I see you had a nice bath—or shower?" I said.

He replied, "So they say! I didn't see any of it though."

It was time for Edwin to visit the dentist again. Mainly we were trying to control the plaque build-up on his teeth, which he seemed to develop in abundance those days, so I took him every four months, wanting to avoid problems further on. Of course his inability to brush his teeth properly obviously added to the problem, and it was never an easy task for the nurse or me to brush them for him. In most cases, he'd try to eat the toothbrush, clamping down on it with his teeth, and making it almost impossible to do the job effectively, if at all. At any rate, the four months were up again, and we went off to see the dentist for his regular appointment to have his teeth cleaned. The dental assistant was very friendly as usual, and asked Edwin what we were going to do that afternoon after his appointment, knowing that we usually made an event of those outings.

"We're going out for a nice lunch in a restaurant." I answered for him.

Turning to Edwin she asked, "And what would you like to have for lunch?"

"Three women!" was his reply.

"Oh!" she said, somewhat surprised at his answer. "Do you think you could handle three women?"

"I'm sure I could do quite nicely!" he replied.

We both had to smile at that.

Once we were seated at the restaurant, the waiter brought us each a glass of water.

Edwin sipped his right away and then said, "I hope you realize this wine is unflavoured!"

Later he asked me, "What was that guy's car?"

"What car?" I asked.

"The car the guy drove us over in," he replied.

"But I drove us over here!" I exclaimed.

"No you didn't! The guy did!"

Realizing the futility of arguing, I just answered his question, "The car was a Grand Am."

"Nice car!" he commented. "If things had gone well I would have been driving one of those myself."

What could I say? It used to be his car!

After awhile he said, "Any idea where our former friends are?"

"What former friends?" I asked.

"The bread and butter type," was his reply.

I then offered to butter some more bread for him, which seemed to be the correct answer.

He responded, "That will do nicely."

After the meal I said, "Wasn't that a delicious meal?"

He replied, "Something like that."

It was such a lovely day weather-wise that I hated to take him home yet so I took him over to Alma's place again, where we enjoyed tea on her patio.

At one point Edwin commented, "I saw a truck load of half-naked women!"

Alma responded with a chuckle, "They weren't half-naked Ed, they were all naked!"

He loved that and grinned from ear to ear!

He also made another comment at Alma's place, one that had become a favourite saying of his for a while, and I'm quoting it verbatim.

"I need a blow job!" he'd say, while reaching for his handkerchief.

Literally very true, of course, but not exactly appropriate, and certainly rather embarrassing when he'd say it in public; especially so, after he discovered the *"neat little zippered pocket"* in the front of his trousers and started stuffing his handkerchief in there. I can't tell you the number of times he had me blushing—and I don't blush easily!

Rather than participating in a two-way conversation, on one of his typical, more talkative days he would carry on with "one-liners" such as the following.

When we couldn't find any of his handkerchiefs one day I gave him a face cloth to use.

Taking it from me, he said, "I had these papers for over two years now, and I never used them."

Most of the time there was nothing I could say in response.

Then he commented, "I hope everything comes out of these boxes alright, "cause everyone will be looking at us."

Later, he said suddenly, "As soon as we get to the highway cut-off, I'll know where we are to the point."

Everything he said seemed to come out of nowhere, and I enjoyed many such one-way conversations with him over time.

When he sneezed one day I handed him a Kleenex.

He said, "What's the drill?"

"Use it to wipe your nose," I said.

"Why?" he asked.

"Because you sneezed," I replied.

He just said, "Oh!"

Ordinarily I didn't let him use Kleenex any more, as he'd taken to eating them and would choke, making it necessary for me to forcibly remove the soggy wad from his mouth. Also, even before that, when he used to have a box of tissues in his room, he'd use the entire box in one evening, wrapping up all his belongings. Thus we graduated to handkerchiefs, even though they had a habit of disappearing as well. However, that day I couldn't find any of his handkerchiefs so I had to give him a Kleenex, but made sure to watch him carefully.

I can't believe the number of handkerchiefs he would go through—it seemed like I was constantly buying them, a dozen at a time—but they always managed to disappear eventually and I'd have to purchase more. Socks were another item that continually disappeared, so I bought a lot of those too. One other item I purchased on numerous occasions—too many to remember—were sweat suits with zippered tops. They didn't disappear, but the zippers kept breaking so I'd have to buy another set. It was still cheaper than buying the jackets separately, besides which, after a few washings the pants would become too short for his long legs, so I didn't mind. Another hat for me—*purchasing agent*! Of course, Edwin didn't recognize that hat. He just accepted everything as his due.

As a fund-raising stunt, Leisureworld had a pie-throwing event, using some of the "important personnel" from the nursing home on the receiving end of the pies. (Victims, actually!) The manager of the Home, a well endowed, attractive lady, sat in the middle, flanked by some of her section heads. I bought a pie (all cream) for Edwin to throw, and I think he really enjoyed it. Of course, he had to see someone else doing it first, but then he took his pie and headed straight for the lady manager. The only thing is, he didn't actually throw his pie at her, just walked right up to her and— almost in slow motion—put the pie right in her face! What a mess! She was a good sport though, her only comment being, "This is like Chinese torture!"

During his second year at the nursing home I bought a wheelchair for Edwin. It was nothing fancy, just a standard model, and though not cheap, it was the least expensive one I could find. This enabled me to take him outdoors for walks in the fresh air. Since he could no longer navigate the uneven surfaces outside, it made it possible for him to enjoy many lovely outings, which would otherwise have been impossible. It also allowed me to continue taking him downstairs for the various activities, which he enjoyed, or if not, at least it provided a diversion for him. At any rate, the chair I bought served him well until such time as he required a wheelchair full-time; necessitating the purchase of a better one, specially made for him and very expensive but comfortable for more prolonged use. At that time I donated the first one to the Home for others to use and enjoy. Until that time though, it proved to be a very worthwhile purchase and gave him much pleasure, enabling him to get about with greater mobility.

Another activity at Leisureworld included summer barbecues with entertainment, so I would take Edwin in his new wheelchair. He enjoyed them thoroughly, even if he couldn't figure out what to do with his hamburger. Taking it in his hands, he'd tear it all apart, making a complete mess of it, so I'd have to feed it to him piece by piece. He really enjoyed the ice cream though, so I'd give him mine as well. You'd have thought I'd given him a million dollars! He loved ice cream! All summer long they would hold those barbecue lunches, complete with great entertainment, every Friday at noon and I tried to take Edwin each week whenever I could, at least until I started working. As it was, it would have been an impossibility without the wheelchair, both in getting him downstairs, and in controlling him during the festivities, so that gave me another reason to be grateful for my purchase. That way too, I didn't have to worry about him wandering off, or falling and injuring himself, especially when I'd have to leave him to collect his food.

One day I found Edwin with a very bruised left hand. I asked him what he had done to hurt it.

He replied, "I can't 'splain it in this consideration that I can 'splain it."

So much for getting an answer to my question! Guess I'll never know, as none of the nurses seemed to be able to explain it either. Obviously it happened when no one was looking. Even with twenty-four hour care it's impossible to be watching all the time.

Once again I found Edwin wandering the halls in a state of undress. Of course that's a matter of interpretation, as he thought himself to be well dressed. He was wearing only his undershirt and under-shorts, with an extra undershirt around his hips resembling a skirt. What a sight he was too! He wore his socks as well, with his shoes on the wrong feet. Apparently he'd refused to get washed and dressed, and had forcibly ejected the nurse who had tried to accomplish it. When I asked him what he was up to, he stated his intention of leaving the facility.

I just said, "Fine, but you'll have to get dressed first. You can't go outside like that!"

That was all it took! He allowed the nurse and myself to lead him to his room and we dressed him between us. Of course I had to take him out after all that—a promise is a promise, even in those circumstances—so I took him for a nice walk in his wheelchair.

One day my husband greeted me, very matter-of-factly, with the news that he was going to kill me!

"Whatever for?" I asked.

"For making a fool of me," he answered.

"How did I do that?" I questioned.

"By taking me to all these places that don't exist!" was his reply.

Whatever that meant! I certainly didn't know where he was coming from but, fortunately, he soon forgot about it.

His following dental appointment was in cooler weather, so I dressed Edwin in his old, comfortable, leather jacket before going outside. As usual, we went out for lunch after the dentist. We sat in a booth at the restaurant and Edwin somehow became convinced that we were on an airplane going to Florida. Thus, on leaving our table, he was sure we'd arrived in Florida and were deplaning. Coming out of the restaurant—cum-airport—afterwards, Edwin suddenly noticed his leather coat, commenting on it.

"This is a nice coat," he said. "I don't know why I never bought myself one of these!"

He'd had that coat for years!

When my husband wanted to use his handkerchief he'd look everywhere for it, even opening his fly. One day when I handed him a new handkerchief, he used it and then commenced to roll it up neatly and carefully, as was his usual habit, but then he tried to put it into his fly. (He loved that neat little pocket.) Trying to break him of the habit of using that particular location, I directed his hand into the pocket of the sweat top he was wearing. However, instead of entering the pocket, his hand went right inside the jacket to the fleece lining.

Stroking the soft fleece, his whole face lit up as he exclaimed, "Oh, I like that!"

I realized that day how important *touch* and *feeling* were for Alzheimer's patients, and following that incident I started bringing Edwin some soft, stuffed animals for him to hold, which he seemed to enjoy. On many occasions after that, I'd find him sitting quietly on his chair and stroking one of the soft toys quite happily, sometimes for hours on end.

One day I arrived to find him perched on a chair in the hallway, gently stroking a huge, live, white rabbit, which was sitting in his lap. Luna had brought in several animals for Activation that day and had assigned the rabbit for Edwin to hold. His face radiated a glow of utter rapture as he sat there stroking the bunny's back, and it seemed to me that he was thoroughly enjoying the experience. However, when I commented on it he was quick to deny my impression.

"I hope you realize I'm only doing this under duress?" he proclaimed, stoutly.

Maybe he was—but he certainly appeared to be enjoying it nonetheless! He was also in no hurry to hand it back to Luna.

For his birthday one year, I bought Edwin a toy camera. Knowing his penchant for cameras, and that he had been a photographer, the staff at Leisureworld had recommended I try it. He seemed quite fascinated with the camera, turning it over and over in his hands, so I thought maybe we'd found a winner. I encouraged him to try taking a photograph of something and showed him where to push the red button to take a (pretend) picture. However, he balked at that. He absolutely refused to push the red button.

"Oh I can't do that!" he exclaimed.

"Why not?" I asked, puzzled.

"Oh no," he said, "It's far too dangerous! That's the top one of the whole thing!"

I have no idea what he was afraid of. Maybe it related to his years in the Air Force as an aerial photographer, flying reconnaissance flights over enemy territory, where they had been admonished not to fire their guns at any cost. Their orders were to take the pictures and get out fast, shooting only as a final measure in self-defense. Perhaps the button to fire the ammunition was red? Who knows?

At any rate, the camera disappeared the next day— never again to surface—so I didn't have to worry about it for long. So much for that idea!

Every Christmas, Leisureworld also sponsored a Christmas Tea, another beautiful occasion with a lovely buffet, great entertainment, and an elegant, festive atmosphere. I was always very impressed at the lengths they would go to, making those occasions so special for the patients and their families and friends. In my estimation they went "above and beyond," and

I appreciated all their efforts to accomplish a friendly, happy, homey atmosphere for all concerned at the nursing home. I'm sure there are many other lovely nursing homes to be found as well, but for Edwin and myself, I couldn't have chosen better and I will always be grateful to all that laboured there, the entire staff included, for each contributed in their own special way to make it such a wonderful place.

Sitting with Edwin at the Christmas Tea, we were joined by Gema, the new head nurse from Edwin's floor.

"Hi Edwin!" she greeted him warmly. "Who is this nice lady beside you?"

I was amazed and pleased to hear him answer, "She's my wife."

However, my pleasure was very short lived as he went on to say, "My wife will be arriving shortly."

His moments of lucidity by then were very rare—and extremely short.

Edwin's third Christmas in the nursing home, the nurses asked me specifically not to take him out for Christmas dinner. They were having so much trouble with him whenever he returned that they were afraid of what he might do, especially after a prolonged absence. They explained to me that Alzheimer's patients eventually do tend to settle in to their new environment, even if it doesn't always appear to be the case. However, taking them out of their familiar surroundings, other than for short jaunts, tends to disorient them and can prove very unsettling, which seemed to be the stage Edwin had reached by then.

They felt it was better to leave him in a regular, scheduled environment, than to upset him unnecessarily. I was disappointed but I could certainly see the wisdom in their request so I complied. It was an extremely lonely Christmas without him though, and a very sad one for me, as was every Christmas by then. The Home did their best to make it as nice as possible, providing a lovely turkey dinner on Christmas day, with all the trimmings, but it just wasn't the same, of course. However, we also enjoyed several Christmas parties, complete with entertainment and gifts for all the patients, sponsored by various organizations and appreciated by all I'm sure. Nevertheless, those days Christmas was not something I looked forward to celebrating. It was just another day and a sad one at that.

One evening when I sat with Edwin at dinner I excused myself for a few minutes to fetch something from his room. The nurse came to sit with him while I was gone.

She asked him, "So Edwin, who is the nice lady sitting with you this evening?"

"I have no idea!" was his reply.

He was always glad to see me but he still didn't know who I was. Usually he just thought that I was someone who worked at the "hotel" where he was staying.

Another hat!

Another day he seemed very surprised to see me.

"What are you doing in this part of my household?" he asked, surprise and pleasure evident in his voice.

It was very surprising one day, walking into Edwin's room, to be greeted warmly with a cheery welcome. That certainly was a departure for him—not his usual style at all.

"And how are you doing today, Mrs...Mrs...whatever your name is?" he floundered.

Just another new hat!

Arriving at the nursing home one day, I discovered Edwin walking hand-in-hand with his new lady friend, one of the patients on his floor. When I spoke to him, he turned to her to question my identity. At first she said I was her friend, but then she amended it to say I was her daughter. Another hat? The nurse tried to correct her but to no avail, so I told her not to bother. At first it used to hurt me terribly, when he didn't know me at all, but by then I was used to it. Perhaps it was better that way anyway. It made things a lot easier when he didn't recognize me anymore. At least that way he didn't miss me as much when I had to leave. I was still trying to find the positive note in everything.

One day, on my arrival, I found him holding hands and walking down the hall with yet another lady! (What a fickle-hearted, lady-killer he was!) I took his other hand, encouraging him to come with me to his room where we could visit in private. Unfortunately his new lady friend was most upset, refusing to let go of him, and tagging along with us. When I gently disengaged her hand, at the door of his room, she shouted at us as we retreated into his chamber.

"You won't sleep with me but you'll go to bed with her!" she yelled.

She was jealous!

I had to smile at the implication, even though I was also embarrassed!

Again, another day, I found him down the hall in a state of undress, this time wearing only his diaper, a pyjama top and one shoe. I took him back to his room where the nurse came in to get him washed. While she was busy dressing him, Edwin pointed to me and commented energetically.

"She's gorgeous!" he said.

Well at least it was nice to know he hadn't lost his appreciation for the ladies, even if he didn't recognize them!

When I would leave the nursing home in the evening I'd usually have to wait for the elevator after keying in the secret code. There were several comfortable chairs in the hallway, in front of the nursing station, facing the elevator, and many patients availed themselves of them, especially if they were waiting for a visitor. Some of the conversations I was privy to while waiting for the lift were really quite humorous. In most cases they would be talking about me while I was standing there, commenting on my clothing, my bearing, my appearance, and anything else they could think of at the time. For the most part, though, they all agreed that I was a very nice young girl. I especially like the "young girl" part.

We were visiting in Edwin's room one day when a patient, sitting on one of the chairs in the hallway outside his door, started yelling something over and over. She'd stop for perhaps a minute or two and then start in all over again, going on and on for ages. It really was quite annoying after a while, so it wasn't too surprising to hear Edwin complain about it.

"It's okay," I said. "Just ignore her."

"Well she should stop," he insisted. "Someone should stop her!"

"I know," I said, "but she can't help it. She doesn't realize she's doing it."

Then Edwin said, "Well they have places for people like that. She should be in a nursing home!"

I didn't bother to point out the obvious!

I don't know where he thought he was himself, if not in a nursing home, but I certainly wasn't going to tell him. At that point I figured what he didn't know wouldn't hurt him—or me for that matter. In such cases, "silence was golden!" Besides, it would have been impossible to reason with him, and it would only have upset him or made him angry, and I didn't want to precipitate either situation.

That was definitely one hat I didn't need to wear!

These Wheels Were Meant for Walking

CHAPTER 17

As mentioned in the previous chapter, the time eventually arrived when Edwin required a wheelchair full time. He could no longer be trusted to wander around on his own, as it wasn't safe for him. Over the months I had repeatedly received calls from the nursing home, reporting falls that Edwin had taken, but as time advanced, those calls became more frequent, and the damage to him more extensive. In fact, on one occasion he actually broke his finger, although he didn't seem to be aware of it at the time. I had taken him to the hospital, where we spent hours waiting for service, and then after they put a splint on his finger, he immediately removed it. What a waste of time and effort that was, especially since he didn't seem to be bothered by the break at all.

By that stage Edwin would be catatonic for long periods of time, completely unaware of his surroundings and totally immobile. Whether sitting or standing, it made no difference, as he would freeze in one position, rooted to the spot, immovable. He could stand—or sit—like that for hours on end, motionless, suspended in time, and completely out of it. However, when those sessions took him while standing, all the blood would rush to his feet, causing them to become swollen and immobile as well. Thus, when he did "return to earth," as it were, his feet could not support him, and he would lose his balance and fall at his first attempt to take a step. Those tumbles on the hard, cement tiles were becoming a concern to me, as well as to the nursing staff, as they could not be watching him constantly. This prompted them to commit Edwin to his wheelchair most of the time. His safety was paramount, as well it should be, and they could no longer take the chance of his hurting himself so they stated unequivocally that he was now required to be in a wheelchair whenever he was out of bed.

One day he took one of his tumbles while I was assisting him to walk to the bathroom. In trying to stop him from falling, I ended up flying over top of him, breaking my arm in the process. A couple of the patients, strolling past our room at the time, just laughed to see me rolling on the floor, but walked on by, totally unaware of our predicament or our need for help. I'm sure I must have looked rather hilarious, to say the least; I was certainly embarrassed. However, at that moment I was more concerned with my husband.

Unfortunately, my attempt to keep him from falling had been unsuccessful, but I think I managed somehow, to lessen the impact of his fall. At least he didn't hit his head. In fact, he landed on the floor in a sitting position, but with a decided list to the right, remaining in that same, listing posture for quite some time. Since no one came when I called for help, I picked myself up and went down the hall to look for a nurse, as I was unable to lift Edwin off the floor by myself. Even without the broken arm I wouldn't have been able to manage it, as he was unable to offer any help, and lifting him was like trying to lift a dead weight. It required two people.

When I finally returned, with two nursing assistants to help me, we found him in exactly the same position as I'd left him, still sitting straight-backed on the floor, and leaning at a good 45-degree angle to the right. He was frozen to the spot and absolutely catatonic. He had no idea what had happened to him and was totally oblivious to his surroundings. That incident completely unnerved me, as I found it impossible to understand how a person could be so unaware of such a traumatic event, but from that day on I never attempted to take Edwin to the washroom—or anywhere, for that matter—on my own again.

That was another lesson I learned the hard way, as I seemed to learn all my lessons, but it also marked a further decline in his condition, as far as I was concerned at least. Previously I had been able to do so many things for him, but not any more. Now I had to depend totally on others to minister to his daily needs.

As it happened, that particular incident occurred just before I was to begin working full time again, so my return to the work force was delayed by a month, while my arm healed. That gave me more time to be with my husband, but it also helped me to appreciate the fact that since I was unable to care for any of his physical requirements anymore, he didn't need me at the same level as before, making it easier for me to face leaving him for my new employment during the day.

When I bought Edwin's first wheelchair I applied to the ADP (Assistive Devices Program) for help in purchasing it. They sent out a representative to assess him but turned down my request.

The reason?

Because, according to them, he did not need to be in a wheelchair full-time!

That was quite true, of course, so I didn't question it. Understanding their reasoning, I accepted their decision and bought him a chair myself, albeit the least expensive one I could find, just a standard wheelchair that was not overly comfortable.

The second time, however, since he was required to be in a chair permanently, I figured there would be no problem. I was wrong! Again they turned me down! This time they said that I should have applied for their help earlier, *before he needed the chair full time*, while he could have operated it by himself. The fact that they had turned me down, *because* he didn't need it then, was of no consequence to them. However, this time I refused to accept "No" as an answer!

The nurses on his floor, Luna in Activation, and myself, all worked prodigiously in training Edwin to use the chair on his own. Of course he was unable to "drive" it, using the normal method of turning the wheels by hand, but we were able to encourage him to use his feet to propel himself along, getting him to follow us down the hallway quite successfully. When he became fairly proficient in his new mode of travel, I reapplied to the ADP, but then I also arranged with Gema, the head nurse, to let me know ahead of time when the representatives from the ADP were coming, so I could plan to be there as well for the assessment process. It was a good thing too!

That day I arrived at the Home an hour before the ADP people were scheduled to be there, only to discover that they had come early and were about to leave. In fact, they had already declared Edwin unfit—again—to qualify for a chair. I was most upset and demanded to know why, so they explained. Apparently they had simply gone into Edwin's room and told him that he was to go out into the hall, propelling his current chair, and then turn around and return to his room again. Since he was incapable of understanding what they were telling him to do, he was unable to comply with their instructions. Thus, they deemed him ineligible. I was very upset and demanded a re-examination, trying to explain to them that the reason he didn't follow their instructions was because he couldn't understand them.

"Don't you know," I explained, somewhat exasperated, "he has Alzheimer's disease! He can't understand multiple instructions! He can only understand one thing at a time, and even then it has to be spoken loudly and clearly."

So saying, I walked out into the hallway myself and called Edwin to come to me. He came, walking his feet as we'd taught him, propelling his chair out to where I was standing in the hall! Then I walked back into his room and told him to come to me once more. Again he came!

"There!" I said, turning to the ADP people. "He *can* do it! He *just* needed to *understand* what you wanted from him."

There was no question after that demonstration! He got his chair—and a beautiful chair at that! The nurses and I were ecstatic, and I was very grateful once again for all their help and encouragement.

I learned a valuable lesson that day. All too often we need to fight for what we want and need—and believe in—in this life. In our case, the personnel from the ADP really didn't understand the situation because they couldn't relate to our particular circumstances. They had never been in our shoes and were therefore unable to see things from our perspective. Thus they made their decision by judging the situation as they thought it should be, and not on how it was in actuality. I am only grateful for their willingness to realign their thinking; enlarging their perception, and reassessing their value system. Hopefully, our experience might help to pave the way for others in similar circumstances in the future.

Ultimately they came through for us and provided us with a wonderful wheelchair, much better than anything I could have afforded, and one that served Edwin well for a long time. With their help I only had to pay for a quarter of the cost of the chair, while the ADP subsidized the rest. (It was still a lot of money, as it was a very expensive chair, but worth every penny it cost me.) I could never have bought such a marvellous chair without their help, and I was very thankful for organizations such as that one, which are in place to help people in similar situations.

As for Edwin, the new chair opened up a whole new world for him, as he could now navigate the halls once more, no longer confined to his room all the time, or his bed. Also, and most important, the new chair was very comfortable for him and he was able to sit in it for hours at a time without damaging his back and bony hips—or his backside! Until that time, Edwin had been limited to being in his room or the lounge for a large part of the day, unable to wander the corridors on his own, and thereby no longer able to enjoy any sense of freedom whatever, even if somewhat limited at best. As well, since his old chair had not been built for comfort, or intended for long periods of use, he was required to spend more time in bed, in order to alleviate the pain of sitting in his chair too long. Thus his new wheelchair offered many benefits, allowing him to enjoy more time among the other patients, rather than being confined to his own company.

After that I took advantage of every day the weather cooperated, taking Edwin outside as much as possible for long walks, visits to the coffee shop or an ice cream parlour, or for a picnic in the park. As well, it enabled me to wheel him over to a nearby restaurant for a good meal, a treat he really enjoyed. Sometimes his son would go along as well and he'd push his dad in the new chair, pretending to be a chauffeur, or a travel guide, or even a bus driver, calling out the stops. Edwin loved that and would laugh along with us, delighting in the repartee.

On those outings he would eat a hearty meal, usually devouring even more than I did, and appearing to enjoy it. However, he still had a problem with eating, most of the time, and needed steady encouragement. He'd eat a little bit and then forget what he was supposed to be doing. Either that or he'd just get tired— or lazy. Then I would have to feed him, until he'd "remember" how to do it himself, and start eating his own food again, though not always. At any rate, he thoroughly enjoyed the restaurant food, and the outing, as well as the company, and it was always a pleasure to see him eating so well and enjoying himself. That was our reward.

The many wonderful features of the wheelchair also facilitated my taking Edwin out more often, as it was lightweight and fully collapsible. As such, it also folded flat, fitting nicely into the trunk of my car with relative ease. That feature alone was a real help to me—and my poor aching back! In fact, the folding chair fit into the car a lot easier than did Edwin, who refused to fold as easily, much to my chagrin at times. Trying to get *him* into the car had become quite a feat by then. Over time I had found that the easiest way to seat him was to turn him around with his back to the door, enabling him then to sit down into the car. All he had to do was bend his legs and sit down. After that I'd lift his legs and swing him around to face the front, before doing up his seat belt, and we'd be on our way. However, as time advanced and the disease took its toll on him, Edwin lost the ability to understand the concept of bending his knees to sit. Whether trying to seat him in the car or in a chair, it made no difference. He'd remain ramrod stiff, and lean straight back without bending his knees or his legs, and I'd end up holding all his weight, as I held on to his hands.

I'd keep saying to him, "Bend your knees! Bend your knees!" but to no avail.

He'd just fall backward, stiff as a board, and I'd have to pull him up again before he hit his head. It was extremely frustrating! One day, after I'd told him to "bend his knees" several times, he actually did bend one of them—but not in the way I'd expected. As he stood before me, he lifted one leg, bending his knee straight up in front of him, while standing like a flamingo on the other. It was hilarious really, and I ended up laughing so hard, I cried!

The next time I took him to visit Alma, he was on his best behaviour, although he dozed off for a while after tea. However, before leaving he began ranting and raving about the terrible place he lived, claiming that they "stripped the people naked and then got out the whips and beat them!" Of course we both knew it wasn't true, so we just let it go. As it was though, some of the things he would say in public from time to time could be quite embarrassing, and easily misconstrued by others. I was just glad there was no one else to hear that story. Where did he get all his fantasies? I'm sure I don't know.

It became apparent, as the months passed, that Edwin's weight was slowly dropping, along with his acuity, not rapidly, but by a slow, steady rate. He did eat, although not a great deal, but I tried to encourage him as much as possible in that regard and would bring him tasty snacks to supplement his intake. One day I asked him at lunchtime if he was hungry for his lunch.

He replied, "Well they have four or five guys working on it, to get the hardware out of the way."

So much for answers!

On one of our walks outside, with Edwin in the wheelchair, the subject of age arose as Edwin asked me how old I was, thinking me to be still a young girl. (I only wish!)

"Are you still in school?" he asked me.

"No I'm not," I replied. Then I countered by asking, "How old are you?"

"Around forty, I think," was his reply.

"That's pretty good!" I remarked.

"Not in Britain it isn't!" was his response.

When we returned to his room after the walk, Edwin commented on how fast the movers had brought his furniture to the new place. He thought he'd gone to a completely new home! However, the main thing was, he liked his new place and was quite impressed with it, so I didn't bother trying to disabuse him. As long as he was happy!

Early in the new year, the nursing home experienced a flu outbreak and shut down the Home to visitors for three weeks. Fortunately Edwin did not get sick, but I was beside myself with worry, not being allowed to visit him, and wondering how he was and if he was missing me. Phoning every day to check the status of the closure, and to inquire about my husband, I felt the three weeks seemed like months before it opened again. I stewed the entire time, thinking that poor Edwin would be sure I'd deserted him, and I dreaded having to face him my first day back, wondering what his response might be. Would he be angry with me, or disappointed, that I hadn't been there for him? I needn't have worried, however! He hadn't missed me at all. In fact, he didn't even know I hadn't been there! So much for feeling needed!

For a while after that, I even questioned my own motives in going to the Home every day, wondering if I'd only been doing it to soothe my own conscience, but then I remembered that I had made a difference for him, and knew I could again. It was still a shock to me at the time, realizing that he was now living in his own private world, a world in which I could come or go but never really existed. However, I also came to recognize the fact that it was a blessing as well, for I no longer needed to feel the pressure of *having* to be at the home every day, unable to give in to my own pain or illness or days of incapacity. Now I could do some things for myself also—without feeling guilty. In fact, I had been struggling with a very sore back for some time, having injured it on several occasions in the past, while helping Edwin in and out of his chair or the car. Now if need be, I could justify my not going to visit him when my back was just too painful.

Thus it helped to ease the pressure of responsibility for me, a burden I'd carried much too long by then. In fact, I even went one step farther and planned a two-week visit to my brother and his wife in Nova Scotia. I desperately needed a break and visiting them was something I'd wanted to do for a long time. I enjoyed the trip immensely, especially knowing that Edwin was in good hands and no longer depending on me, and also relieved of the fear that Edwin would think I had deserted him. The rest did me a world of good and on my return I was far better able to cope, for having had the break. From that time on I made a point of spending fewer hours at the nursing home each day, (not feeling guilty if I missed a day here and there) and more time doing things I needed to do for my self and my own well-being.

Time seemed to stand still during those weeks and months while Edwin was in the nursing home, but still it turned into months and years, as one summer after another would come and go. I loved the summer and all the accompanying outside events that were organized for the patients at Leisureworld. Again, the wheelchair was a wonderful benefit and made it possible for me to take Edwin to the many activities and outings offered during the nice weather. It made me happy too, being able to treat him to all those special occasions sponsored by the Home, which we could not have done without the chair. The wheelchair was worth every cent it cost me and I continued to be thankful for having been able to acquire it at last.

Edwin remained much the same during the years that followed; once he had reached that stage, his condition becoming neither worse nor better. At times he would seem to coast along for extended periods, showing little change or deterioration at all. Then, almost overnight, he would regress, sometimes quite rapidly, falling to another plateau where he'd level out again, albeit at a lower level of capability than before. Thus he appeared to regress by degrees or stages, interspersed with long periods of relative stability, before dropping to yet another level in the process of debilitation.

For myself that time seemed interminable, and I thought it would never end. I tried so hard to be happy and positive around my husband, but as soon as I'd get into the car to drive home at night, the tears would start to flow. I couldn't help it! Many an evening I could hardly navigate the route home, as the tears would blur my vision, and I worried that one day I would have an accident if I continued like that. Each day I'd try to tell myself that tomorrow would be better, simply because it couldn't be any worse, but I could never quite convince my heart. Those were lonely days for me. In fact

I don't think I've ever felt so alone in my life, as I did those long weeks, and months, and years, while my husband languished in the nursing home.

Another dark cloud began to loom on the horizon during those days and I realized that very soon it too would need to be addressed. It was very expensive keeping my husband in the nursing home, especially in a private room, as well as having to maintain my own living expenses, and I knew that sooner or later I was going to have to make some changes. The longer Edwin remained in the Home, the more crucial my financial burden became, until at last it became apparent that I would have to sell the condo and find less expensive accommodations for myself. Also, since Edwin had become unaware of his surroundings by that time, it seemed less important to keep him in a private room. Thus I applied to have him moved from his private room to a ward. It was a very difficult decision to make, but I felt the time had come to make that move. In fact, I thought it might be prudent to have him in a room with someone else, to avoid the possibility of his having an accident and not being found soon enough. At least with a room-mate there would be another person to alert the nurses or call for help. However, even after making the decision, I found his name had merely been added to the end of a very long waiting list, and it was a full year before the move actually took place.

Another distressing possibility was presented to me at that time. I say "distressing" because for me the course of action was not an option, it was not something I would even consider, but for some I realized it could be a matter of necessity. The course suggested to me by others involved with spouses in the nursing home, was to apply for a "legal separation" from my spouse, thereby separating my finances from his, enabling each of us to declare separate incomes. By doing that it would have made it possible for Edwin to qualify for an extra subsidy from the government, to help defray the costs of the nursing home to an even greater extent. I knew people who had done just that and were benefiting from it. However, I could not bring myself to consider such a step. I'm not condemning those who did—not at all—but each person has to do what is best for them, and their conscience, and I just could not follow such a course. It certainly had its advantages, for some more than others, but the down side for many is that they also lose control over the choice of treatment for their loved ones, a choice I refused to relinquish. Thus I could neither recommend nor condemn that course of action. I leave the choice to others to do what is best for them and their loved ones in their own situation.

Eventually circumstances forced me to sell the condo and I moved into a small, rental apartment in order to give myself time to decide what area I'd like to settle into permanently, which I did nine months later. As well, after months of sending out numerous resumes, I finally accepted a secretarial job, working Monday to Friday in order to pay the bills, which were beginning to mount by that time. I was very grateful to have been able to find work and dedicated myself to doing the best job I could for my new employers. As well, I continued to visit the nursing home regularly, evenings and weekends. Fortunately, by that time Edwin didn't seem to be aware of my reduced visiting hours, but still I couldn't bear to forsake him, and I spent as much time as possible by his side.

Some months after I started working Edwin became catatonic the majority of the time, neither greeting me on my arrival, nor acknowledging my presence while there, so I'd just sit down beside him and start telling him about my day, or reading to him from my latest book interest. Sometimes I'd get a modicum of response from him, but more often than not he'd just sit there, silent and staring.

Sometimes I'd ask myself, why am I doing this? Why do I bother coming, when he doesn't even know I'm here? But then I'd remember stories I'd heard, about people in similar situations, or coming out of comas, and saying they remembered people talking to them, so I'd carry on, depressed and lonely at times, but still determined to do what I could.

During that stage as well, Edwin would often take a turn for the worse, coming down with pneumonia (a common ailment among inactive patients), or falling out of bed, or whatever else might occur, and the nursing home would call me to say he'd been rushed to hospital. Those times I'd race to the hospital, where I'd usually find him lying on a stretcher in the hallway, where he'd remain for half the night, until someone would finally attend to him. Then when the emergency was pronounced to be over, we'd wait another few hours for the ambulance to pick him up again and return him to the Home. Those nights I'd be lucky to get two or three hours of sleep, if any, before having to leave for work the next day. (Interestingly enough, those episodes never seemed to happen on a weekend, only on working days! Murphy's law, I guess!)

Thus the days passed, turning into weeks and months, as I continued to watch him slowly deteriorating before my eyes. It was demoralizing, for myself as much as for him, but I continued to do what I could, which didn't seem like much, but there really wasn't very much anyone could do any more, except to try and keep him comfortable. I also continued to wheel him about in his wheelchair, just to give him a change of view, if nothing else, and carried on taking him to all the entertainments provided by the Home. He could no longer walk his own chair but I still determined to keep him "mobile" as long as possible, being rewarded for my efforts the odd time, by a sudden glimmer in his eye, or an unexpected smile, briefly lighting the contours of his face. That was all I needed! That was my reward and I treasured those moments out of all proportion.

Did I do all those things for myself as much as for my husband? Perhaps so! I really couldn't tell you what motivated me exactly, as it was a combination of things, including love and pity and a strong sense of duty. However, I just knew that I had to do all I could to give my husband some quality of life, some reason to keep on living, because I wasn't ready to lose him yet either. He was also *my* reason for living, and as long as he needed me, I needed to be there for him.

Going Home

CHAPTER 18

I was going home and I was excited! Home for me, on that particular day, referred to my daughters' homes in Manitoba. Two lovely daughters, their husbands, and seven grandchildren were looking forward to my visit and it was an exciting time for all of us. It had been several years since I'd last been out west, so the trip was long overdue, and I couldn't wait to see them. My bags were packed and ready to go, and all that remained was one last day at work. My flight was scheduled to leave very early on Saturday morning, and not wanting to work late on Friday evening, I stayed very late at the office on Thursday evening in order to get all my work completed before my vacation. Thus it was after midnight when I finally reached home.

Arriving home tired, but excited about my forthcoming trip, I was dismayed to be greeted by a succession of blinking red lights on my answering machine. Now what?

Since my telephone seldom rang anymore, except for emergencies, I was assailed by a feeling of apprehension: Had Edwin had another fall? What about my daughters? Had something happened to one of them? Was the trip being called off or were they calling to confirm my flight? Of course, that must be it! Nothing to worry about! My mind reeled with questions before I was able to get my emotions under control. Once I calmed down, realizing it was far too late to call anyone back at that hour anyway, I removed my coat and poured myself a glass of pop, before settling down to listen to my messages.

I was wrong! It had nothing to do with my daughters at all—or my trip out west. It was Edwin! He hadn't had a fall either—not this time! There were several frantic calls from the nursing home to the effect that Edwin had been diagnosed with pneumonia and rushed to the hospital around nine o'clock that evening—while I was still at the office! The hospital had phoned as well, to inform me that my husband had been admitted and to let me know in which ward he was located.

Thus began for me a sleepless, four-night-and-day vigil at the hospital, and a cancelled visit to my family out west.

He was comatose when I arrived, and remained that way throughout the long vigil. That night, however, the nurse on duty assured me there was nothing wrong with him, except that they couldn't get any response from him. She asked me about his condition and I told her that such a lack of response was not unusual for him as he had Alzheimer's disease. She then informed me, rather curtly I might add, that the nursing home had sent him there, stating on his chart that he had pneumonia, but she herself saw no evidence of it, since he was neither coughing nor suffering from a runny nose. (Those were her exact words.) In fact, she even went on to say that she didn't know why they had admitted him, since he'd probably just be sent home the next day. Her entire attitude was one of annoyance, obviously irritated at the nursing home for having sent him there in the first place. Nevertheless, I was somewhat heartened by her assessment of the situation, feeling that his condition wasn't as serious as I had first thought. She also insisted that I needn't remain there, but I resisted the temptation to leave, just in case, opting instead to settle down at the hospital for the night. However, in the light of her unofficial diagnosis, I decided not to phone Edwin's son until the next morning, since it obviously wasn't an emergency; rather than give him a wakeful night for nothing. I just wanted to be there myself in case he woke up, confused or frightened by his new surroundings.

As it was, he'd already been rushed to the hospital on several other occasions, only to be returned to the nursing home with no major trauma, and I had no reason to expect this situation to be any different. However, having suffered through those fruitless emergency visits to the hospital with him many times, I understood how traumatic they could be for him, further upsetting him and only adding to his confusion and disorientation, so I wanted to be there for him, to help him through it once again. Even though he didn't know who I was, he still needed someone with him who cared for him, someone who was able to calm him down, and imbue him with some sense or feeling of security in the midst of all his confusion. Though I was unknown to him as a person, somewhere deep inside him, I still think he recognized my touch.

His son arrived at the hospital shortly after I called him the following morning; also worried but somewhat reassured by my recounting the night nurse's comments on his father's condition. That turned out to be a long morning for us, as we waited a prohibitive length of time for the doctor to come. When he still had not arrived by noon, and since the nurses were unable to tell us when he would arrive—even to the point of it being afternoon or evening—we finally decided to go for a much-needed coffee. However, on returning from the cafeteria not ten minutes later, we discovered to our dismay that the doctor had already been there. We had just missed him! I was very upset and asked the nurse to try paging him, only to be informed that she had no idea if he was still in the hospital. Not willing to accept her answer, I insisted that she *try* at least, and she finally agreed to do so. Some time later we were greatly relieved when the nurse returned to our room to say that the doctor was on the phone and would like to talk to me. At last!

The news was not good!

Still in shock, I relayed it to his son. According to the doctor, Edwin's condition was very bad! He had pneumonia in the bottom of both lungs (double pneumonia) and there was no chance of survival.

In the doctor's own words, "It's just a matter of time!"

Of course Edwin's son was just as shaken by the news as was I, and we simply hugged each other and cried. However, after a while we had to face the reality of the situation and do what we could for Edwin, even if just to keep him comfortable.

Unexpectedly, an hour later the doctor I had spoken to on the phone returned to Edwin's room, stating that he wanted to talk to me personally, face to face. What he said was brutally honest but also, I am convinced, prompted by caring concern, both for Edwin and for myself. Reiterating the certainty that my husband had no chance for survival, he advised withholding any further medication, which was only adding to his discomfort and would simply prolong his suffering, suggesting instead that they administer only morphine to keep him as comfortable as possible. In other words, he strongly recommended reverting to palliative care, in order to do everything possible to alleviate his pain, while allowing him to die a natural, but relatively painless death. He also went on to explain that Edwin had entered a comatose state from which he would never return, as that part of his brain was lost beyond repair, emphasizing again that for him it was just a matter of time. There was nothing more they could do—except try to make him comfortable.

We received the doctor's prognosis in absolute shock! However, we also realized ourselves that in his present condition, Edwin was not really living—just existing—and to force him to go on any longer than necessary in such a state would be cruel and selfish. We certainly didn't want him to suffer any more, so of course we agreed to the doctor's recommendation.

Thus continued the vigil, with my sitting up with him through the long nights, and his son coming over in the morning, allowing me to go home for a shower and change of clothing, before returning to the hospital. I tried lying down for a sleep while at home that first day, but was unable to turn off my brain, as it were, which seemed to be working overtime, so I gave it up and returned to his bedside right away. Edwin's son was wonderful, caring and supportive, and I really appreciated his strength during those long, trying hours. One of the nurses commented on the fact that Edwin was one of the lucky ones, having family with him throughout the vigil. She went on to say how so many people just die alone, with no one there, and no one to care. How very sad! My heart went out to them. I can't think of anything worse than dying all alone. It's like taking a big trip with no one to see you off—only far, far worse! Such a lonely feeling! It only strengthened my resolve to see Edwin through his journey, to the bitter end.

The nurses were very kind and supportive and brought me a larger chair, which proved to be a lot more comfortable, to use during the long nights at the hospital. Then in the mornings his son would arrive with muffins and coffee for breakfast, and some lunch that his wife had prepared for us. She even came one day to share our vigil with us. As well, the people from my employment were very supportive and kind, telephoning to cheer me up, dropping by to visit, and bringing me little gifts or snacks. So many kind-hearted people did what they could to help me through those dark days, and I appreciated them all, eminently grateful to God for the wonderful friends with which He had blessed me, and humbled by their loving kindness.

There was one interesting change that occurred in Edwin's condition at the hospital. Whereas he would doze most of the time at the nursing home, especially during the last months of his life, his eyes were usually closed, but during his days at the hospital, his eyes were usually open wide. Indeed, only under the influence of the morphine would his eyes close and his laboured breathing take on the normal sound of sleeping. The rest of the time his eyes would remain wide open, unblinking and staring. I learned later that the diminished capacity of the brain cells also impaired the ability to control reflex action such as blinking, twitching or indeed, moving at all. That also explained the gradual stiffening of his limbs, and the atrophying of his muscles, causing him to be unable to straighten his legs or move his hands. However, at the time I found it rather disconcerting, convinced he was trying to communicate with me.

Sometimes involuntary expressions would pass over his face, reflecting fear or even a look of pleading.

When I'd stroke his brow or touch his cheek it would relax him somewhat, and at times I'd almost convince myself that he was looking right at me, pleading with me, recriminating with me for not doing something more to help him. It was heart-wrenching and made me feel even more wretched and guilty and utterly helpless, so much so that I cried and prayed and pleaded with God, begging him to tell me what more I could do to help him! Later Edwin's son admitted to experiencing the same sensation of his father pleading with him too for help, and the accompanying, overwhelming feeling of helplessness, of being unable to do anything to help—outside of being there. Again I learned, some time later, that those expressions we saw from time to time, actually meant nothing but were merely the result of a dying man losing control over his ability to use those muscles. In fact, it's much the same, apparently, as several basic expressions that are reflected on the face of a baby just stretching its muscles. The expressions we saw were entirely attributable to the rapidly diminishing capacity of the brain to control the facial muscles, and were simply muscular twitches, as it were, and commonly inherent in such situations. It was only our intense longing to help that fed our imaginations so devastatingly, making us feel so vulnerable and inadequate. The knowledge was a comfort to me but I don't think I will ever forget that expression of pleading I saw on his face, or my feelings of utter inadequacy during that time. I still have to remind myself that he was comatose and no longer aware of anything. The suffering was mine—and mine alone—not his!

Monday morning dawned and we were still keeping the vigil. When the doctor arrived around noon, he was surprised to find Edwin still alive, having been convinced that his death was imminent on Friday. He informed us however, that there was nothing more they could do for him so they were sending him back to Leisureworld. We were very surprised to hear his pronouncement, but found out later that such a course of action was common practice these days. Rather than having patients die in the hospital, where a shortage of nurses precludes personalized care, they prefer to send them back to the nursing home where they're better prepared to handle it. In fact, in some cases, where it's practical, and the patients are clearly cognizant, they even send them to their own homes to die, in their own beds, and with friends and loved ones standing by.

When we asked how much longer Edwin had to live, the doctor replied, "I have no idea! I didn't expect him still to be here this morning."

That evening Edwin was taken by ambulance and returned to the nursing home, where I saw him settled back into his old room and comfortably tucked into his bed for the night. It was almost a relief, in a way, to be back in familiar territory, with a nursing staff I'd come to know like a family, and I settled in for the long haul, wondering afresh how many weeks or months he would carry on like this. I'd seen it before with other patients, many of whom I'd befriended along the way. I'd watched them slowly decline into a comatose state, never to return to the real world, but lingering on for month after month, while their loved ones suffered in silent agony, hoping against hope for some glimmer of response. I didn't want Edwin to suffer in any way—but I didn't want to lose him either—and in spite of the doctor's pronouncement, I too shared some small thread of hope. He'd lasted this long, so who could say what might or might not happen. Anything was possible—wasn't it? Perhaps he would come out of it. Maybe we would have another chance. I went home that night to sleep for the first time in four days and it did me a world of good. However, I returned to the Home first thing the next morning, still determined to be there for him.

He died that afternoon!

It was an easy death, very calm and peaceful. He just stopped breathing, nothing more. His breathing had been very shallow all day and his last breath was almost imperceptible when it finally stopped. One minute he was there and the next he was gone, leaving his skin with a grey, waxy pallor as the blood slowly drained from his face and hands. His eyes were still open so I gently shut them as I tenderly kissed him goodbye.

He had finally realized his wish; he had gone home!

During the course of his illness, Edwin's recurring theme, when he was still able to talk, was that he wanted to go home. Of course that did not mean his literal home, as even when living there, he was always packing his bag to leave. One of the saddest circumstances for sufferers of Alzheimer's disease is that they are never at home any more. No matter where they are, because of their disorientation, every place to them is strange. My only comfort at that point was in knowing that—finally—Edwin was at home! He was in his eternal home, and all his years of pain and suffering were behind him at last.

I wept, of course, copiously, but I wept for myself as much as for him, for what I had lost—indeed, in reality, had lost a long five years before that moment in time. I wept for the loss of that comfortable complacency I'd found in my life with Edwin, that special bond of togetherness and camaraderie that one shares alone with one's partner in life—my soul mate as it were. All that was gone now, drowned forever in a sea of tears, a river of remorse, and despair for what once had been and would be no more. It was lost, beyond recovery, and all that remained was the shell of a man and the hollow echo of what once was but could exist no longer.

I can't begin to describe the feeling of complete and abject loneliness that overwhelmed me after that final loss. I was completely devastated. I'd known he was going to die—eventually—and I was even prepared for his death, *but I was not ready*. Even though I had done all the work of preparation for that day, realizing it was inevitable, even to making arrangements and prepaying the funeral, still I was unable to face the reality of that devastating loss. No matter how prepared I was, I was not ready—nor would I ever have been ready! In retrospect I don't think anyone is ever ready, not really, not completely prepared to face the stark reality of loss in all its finality. I know I wasn't! I just felt like I was living on the edge of a chasm, just waiting for the rest of the world to cave in on me. It was completely overwhelming!

Now, it was finally over— all his pain and suffering, all the indignities inherent in that debilitating disease; the inability to perform even the most basic, primal tasks for oneself; all the fear and turmoil engendered by the lessening of comprehension, due to the shrinkage of his brain cells, and the accompanying chaos of confusion, frustration and fear. All of it was over at last! For Edwin it had to be a sweet release, and I was glad for him. Then why was I crying? How selfish could I be? I didn't want him back to suffer longer. Heaven forbid! I cried for him: for what he used to be and for all the good times we'd shared together. I cried for what could never be again! I cried for what we'd lost! I cried for what I'd lost! I cried for me—alone again—with no one to care for, and no one to care for me! It was the final chapter in our book of life! This time, it really was the end!

It was also the end for me, the end of life as I had known it in the past, and the end of a longer vigil than that of the past four days and nights; that vigil which began over five years earlier, when he was first diagnosed with Alzheimer's disease. Now that vigil too was over! What now? Suddenly that question echoed in my mind and I was reeling under the strength of its refrain. *What now*? What *can* I do now? What *should* I do? I felt hopelessly lost, and alone, and completely vulnerable.

The staff at Leisureworld were wonderful, having become like family to us over the past five years since Edwin had arrived there, and they were very kind and supportive, allowing me ample time to grieve, before addressing the practical issues facing them. I phoned Edwin's son as soon as I was able, letting him know his father had gone, and he in turn phoned Alma, who drove right over to be with me and to help me through that devastating experience. Again I was very grateful for her help and support. What a wonderful blessing good friends can be during difficult times. How I thank God continually for the wonderful friends he has given me over the years.

The nursing home contacted the doctor who was required to sign the Death Certificate before they could remove the body, so I had to wait for him to arrive, before phoning the funeral parlour to come pick up Edwin, and I waited there in an agony of restless uncertainly. I was so glad to know that all the details had been pre-arranged with the funeral parlour, as there was no way I could have been able to think clearly at that juncture, but even so the whole experience was overwhelming and I moved as if in a dream— or more aptly, a nightmare. This wasn't happening to me, it couldn't be! I just wanted the pain to stop, but at that moment I was convinced it would never cease. I tried not to think, for to think was to feel, and feeling was just too painful to bear. I didn't want to feel anything right then.

My tears continued to flow and I felt utterly devoid of life itself, devastated and drained. I kept on trying to tell myself that death was a blessing for Edwin, a sweet release for him, and I knew it in my head, but my heart would not yet accept it and I continued to cry for myself.

Even now, committing my feelings to paper has caused more tears to flow but I realize at last—no, I am convinced—that they are now tears of healing, washing over my soul and gradually refreshing my spirit. Time does heal wounds and though some things are never forgotten, their memories become sweeter and less painful with the gentle passing of time. It is human nature to remember the good things, the happy occasions, and over the space of time to forget the pain and suffering that accompanied them. If this were not true, no woman would allow herself to have more than one baby. Believe me, I know that from experience too! However, as time passes, the pain for me is also receding, and thoughts of Edwin now can make me smile at the memory of that sweet, sensitive soul who touched my life for a few precious years.

He had finally gone home at last!

Yellow Roses!

CHAPTER 19

During the last year of Edwin's life, my favourite uncle died and I was present for the visitation and the burial service for him. Then, just a few months later, I had the misfortune to attend the funeral of a very dear friend. I was devastated, having lost two very special people in my life, but at the same time I became aware of the pressing need to make pre-arrangements for such an inevitable circumstance in advance of the occasion. I began to realize just how difficult it was for the grieving families to cope with making all the necessary arrangements, while bearing the burden of grief, and recognized the wisdom of planning ahead so as to lessen the pressure when that time arrived for me. I knew that death was inevitable for Edwin, and that many people were amazed he had continued for as long as he had. In fact, when I mentioned my husband to a friend I hadn't seen for some time, she astounded me by saying, "Edwin? I thought he died long ago!" She was extremely embarrassed of course. Who wouldn't be?

At any rate, I realized the time had come to do something about planning ahead for his demise. Up to that point I had stubbornly refused to acknowledge the need, even to myself, thinking that if I didn't do it, it wouldn't happen. If I didn't plan for his funeral, he wouldn't die. I wonder how many others have felt the same way? I just didn't want to face the truth. However, eventually I had to accept the fact that it was going to happen. I just hoped it wouldn't be too soon.

Not having any idea how to go about putting my thoughts into action, and still wavering about making any decisions, I decided to bring up the subject at the next meeting of the Alzheimer's Support Group, asking their advice on the matter. However, as I sat in the group that evening I found myself tongue-tied. I couldn't do it—I couldn't face it—and the thought of broaching the subject appalled me. Then, just as I had made up my mind to forget it altogether, one of the ladies in our group began speaking to us. June's husband had suffered for many years with Alzheimer's and she had become one of the longest-standing members of our support group. However, her husband had just died, and she wanted to share with us the importance of pre-arranging the funeral. (I couldn't believe my ears! Surely this was fate—or God! Whatever it was, it was just what I needed that evening.) She mentioned how glad she was that she had made arrangements ahead of time for her husband's funeral, stating that she could never have coped otherwise. She went on to urge all of us to consider doing the same, reiterating the fact that it had made a world of difference for her.

Listening to her exhortation was like hearing a voice from heaven for me. I realized she was right and I knew I needed to do the same—before it was too late. Thus it was that the very next day I contacted Ian MacLean, a good friend and a minister, soliciting his advice and expertise. He put me in touch with Richard, from the Trull Funeral Home in Toronto, who was wonderfully helpful and supportive, putting the plans in motion and making it possible for me to pay for their services in bi-weekly amounts over a few months' time. Thus, both the burden of planning for the event, and the financial weight of it were taken care of in due course. I also appreciated the fact that Edwin's son offered to help as well, and between us we managed to pay for all the fundamental arrangements, long before they were required.

When the day ultimately arrived that I needed their services, they were there for me, doing everything necessary—and then some—to ensure that my load was as light as possible, and I will always be grateful. I am just so glad that I finally obeyed my instincts and planned ahead for that contingency as it really did make things so much easier for me in the end. Death is never easy and no one is ever ready for it, but that is all the more reason to be as prepared as possible, for that day will come. As one doctor said to me, "Don't say *if* he dies;

say *when* he dies, for your husband *is* going to die, and you need to face that fact, rather sooner than later."

If the one you love is suffering from Alzheimer's disease, perhaps you also need to face the truth—now. As yet, unfortunately, there is no cure; the disease is inexorable! How much better it is to face it now, and make plans for that inevitable day, than to hold off and have to face it unprepared. I've seen so many people overwhelmed by the sudden burden of death, and all its inherent chores and duties, and I've also seen people circumvented by their grief and despair, allowing others to profit from their misfortune. Don't let that happen to you—or your loved one. Planning ahead allows you to maintain control, when everything around you seems to be out of control, and it will also help to avoid the possibility of others taking advantage of you in your grief.

Take it from someone who knows!

My husband had wanted no funeral service and no viewing. He was adamant about that and I could not disregard his wishes. At the same time though, I also needed closure for myself, and planned to have just a small committal service at the graveside. However, matters grew rather out-of-hand, as so many people from my employment, along with friends and family, wanted to come and pay their respects, that I was at a loss to know how to handle it. Then Richard, the manager of the funeral parlour kindly offered me the use of a lovely room for an informal gathering and "time of remembrance" before going to the cemetery. That proved to be the answer, as well as a real blessing for all who attended. Unexpectedly the weather turned bitterly cold that day, and it had snowed the night before, so it would have been impossible to accommodate many people at the graveside. As it was, that one room actually expanded into two rooms, as more and more people showed up, until we had over 60 people crowded in to share in *A Celebration of Edwin's Life*. It was a beautiful occasion and everyone was delighted with the results, including Edwin's son and myself.

The funeral home had suggested my decorating the room with photos of Edwin, along with some of his photography. I agreed it was a good idea in principle, but approached it with some trepidation, thinking it would be a very difficult task, going through his photos and personal effects. However, to my surprise and delight, the whole exercise was actually quite cathartic instead. I had almost forgotten, during the long struggle with his illness, what a beautiful person Edwin had been. The man I fell in love with originally had become a clouded vision over the last five difficult years with Alzheimer's. Going through his photos inspired the recollection of many pleasant memories, and restored to me a vision of the man I had married, as the real Edwin emerged; not just the shell of the man that he had become. Thus a dreaded task became, in essence, a blessing and a release—a catharsis for my soul. I also wrote a poem about my husband, which was read at the "celebration" of his life, and which I shall include on the last page of this book. The writing of the poem also proved to be an exercise in the process of recovery for me, as happy memories emerged in the forming of the verses.

It was very difficult at the cemetery to say that last goodbye, as we placed our yellow roses on the grave, accompanied by copious tears. Yes, yellow—a vibrant, living colour—representing for us everything that day was not! And yet, in my heart of hearts I knew already that my husband was not being buried in that tomb. Not Edwin, but only his shell—only the container of the man I once knew and loved! He himself continues to live on, in my heart, in my memories, and in all the things I am, and have become, because of him. God allowed us our day in the sun and I shall always be grateful for the time we had together. Now he is in his heavenly home where there is no more sickness, no more pain, and no more sorrow. I could ask no better for him and I can only rejoice that his days of suffering are over at last.

I had not intended to include this chapter when I first conceived of writing about our experiences throughout the years with Alzheimer's disease, but now I realize that it is an integral part of the purpose of the book, to let those experiencing the reality of living with Alzheimer's, and watching a loved one deteriorate, know that they are not alone. Others have gone before them and suffered similar situations. We know what they are going through because we too have travelled that road—and others will again. But there *is* hope and the sun *will* shine again! It's hard to believe it now—I know, believe me, I do know—but the time *will* come and you *will* live again! If I may be allowed, I would like to quote a verse I read in the King James version of the Bible, which has helped me through many a dark day over the past years. It's found in Psalms 30:5 and reads as follows:

"Weeping may endure for a night, but joy cometh in the morning."

How true this is, throughout all our lives. Things always look better in the morning, in the light of day, especially after a good night's sleep. No matter how bad our situation may seem in the darkness of night, when we are tired and worn, the new day brings new hope and new energy to face that day. My long, dark night lasted over five years and it seemed to go on forever. Others may suffer for longer terms, or even shorter periods, but remember this, if nothing else. *A new day is coming*! Hang on to that thought, no matter how hard it is to believe it, when your world seems black, and your faith is not strong enough to pierce the impenetrable darkness. The morning *will* come! A new day *will* emerge from the gloom of night—and you *will* live again!

Now I must begin a new life, not without pain, and not without memories of what might have been, for those are, indeed, the essence of life, and will always be an integral part of mine. However, it will be a life made richer for the experience of the past, and it will be a life lived to the fullest potential. How could I not appreciate the sunshine, having lived through so much rain? How could I not appreciate the spring, after having suffered through such a long, cold winter? How could

I not appreciate the light, having travelled through such a long, dark tunnel? The same must be true for everyone, if we allow it to be so.

"For everything there is a season!" This is a fact of life. Your season will come, maybe not today or even tomorrow, but it will come! Hang on to that thought, plant those seeds, and remember—*you are not alone!*

Epilogue

Following the funeral, my employer offered to give me some time off work in order to allow my bruised emotions to heal. I was totally exhausted, physically and mentally, and needed a break after working at my job and looking after my husband for the past five years, most of which he didn't even know who I was. In that sense I'd already said goodbye to him five years before, but it was still a very long goodbye. Thus, feeling the need to get away from everything, I tried to reinstate my airline ticket for Winnipeg, in order to reschedule my trip out west to visit my daughters. I knew they could be counted on to administer lots of TLC to their grieving mother, and I felt the need of their company more than ever at that time. However, it was not to be and I'm sure you can imagine my disappointment on discovering there were no flights available for over two months; obviously too late for my immediate situation.

Still needing to escape my life for a while, I went to visit a travel agency that I knew specialized in last-minute packages. I asked them to give me something—anything—I didn't care where, as long as it wasn't too expensive and as long as it was warm. Since I was unable to visit my daughters out west, I decided I might as well enjoy a warm climate instead. To my surprise, they suggested Cuba, about which I had only heard negative reports in the past, from friends who had gone there on holidays. However, they assured me it was all changed now and Cuba was a safe and restful place for a vacation. Trusting their recommendation I booked a week in a resort at Varadero, Cuba, and was scheduled to leave four days later. That gave me plenty of time to tie up all the loose ends and take care of the necessary business matters pertaining to the funeral before leaving. As well, it helped to be busy, facing a deadline, and kept my mind off of myself, and my pain. However, even though I was anxious to get away, I just couldn't work up any enthusiasm about my forthcoming holiday. My heart wasn't in it and I wasn't at all excited about going, even though I knew I needed the break. I just felt depressed and lethargic, and packing was the last thing I wanted to do since I couldn't have cared less about what clothing to wear or which things to take with me. It was just another chore that had to be done. Somehow I just couldn't seem to feel strongly about anything right then.

My first three days in Cuba I stayed mostly to myself, feeling overwhelmingly lonely, disorientated and depressed. I cried every day, those first few days, sitting alone in my room every morning and thinking perhaps it had been a mistake to go there at all. Not even changing continents could take away the pain I was feeling, for though I'd left my situation behind, I still had to live with myself. That's what I really wanted to do—leave myself behind—but that was impossible and I knew it. Thus I became convinced that never again would I be happy; no more could I enjoy the gift of life, the love of laughter or the sheer joy of living. My heart was heavy, my life was over, and I could never know happiness again. During those days too, I went for long, vigorous walks along the beach every afternoon, walking for miles and driving myself to exhaustion so I could get some sleep at night. I was depressed and miserable—and incredibly lonely. I didn't want my husband back—at least not the way he was, the person he had become—but I just felt so alone in the world. I wasn't needed anymore and I thought I'd never be happy again.

On the third day, as I was walking along the beach, appreciating the therapeutic massage of the sand undulating under my feet, and the gentle, soothing caress of the sea washing over my toes, I was suddenly surprised out of my reverie by a larger wave that crept up, unnoticed, splashing me from head to foot. It was so unexpected, that sudden invasion of my meditative musings, that I was caught unawares and I laughed out loud. As the realization of what I'd done hit me, I stopped dead in my tracks, amazed at my own soul-stirring response.

I laughed out loud! I couldn't believe it!

I honestly thought I would never laugh again and here I had laughed out loud! Indeed, I had thought myself incapable of laughter, no longer able to feel happiness, to enjoy life, but I was wrong! I had laughed out loud! Suddenly, it was for me as though the heavens had opened and the sun shone through, as the realization of what had happened hit me full force.

I could laugh!

I could feel!

I was alive!

There was life after death!

That day, my walk on the beach, that recalcitrant wave and the sudden drenching, represented for me the water of life, as it were, combining to become a part of the healing process, bringing me back to life; the stepping stone that led me back to the world of the living. From that point on I ceased my retrospection, stopped dwelling on what I had lost, relinquished my tenacious hold on the past, and began to look forward to a new day, a new dawn, and a new beginning. My depression lifted, my vitality returned, and I found myself able to smile again. I could neither change the past, nor could I forget it, and it would inevitably colour my world and my future, but now, however, there was one major difference; now *I could choose the colour*, and just like the roses at Edwin's funeral, I chose the colour yellow—the colour of life!

There will always be those who think my experience by the sea sounds silly and trivial, and perhaps they are right. In fact, it sounds pretty crazy even to me.

However, I thank God for that wave, for getting my attention in such a way that I was able to get my thoughts off of myself and on to the bigger picture. It was a turning point for me, a catharsis as it were, and a purifying of my emotions, that helped to cleanse my heart and soul, giving me the will and the desire to start living again.

Whatever it is for you, embrace it, welcome it, no matter how trifling or puerile it may seem. Never negate what ministers to your emotions and your heart. Just be thankful for the healing and you will find, as I did, that life does go on. It is possible to find happiness again. Just open your heart and it will come—in time. Time is our friend—believe it or not—and time does heal! It may not seem like it today, or even tomorrow, but your new day will come. Life goes on and you *will* live again!

Just bear in mind that those of us who survive the journey with Alzheimer's disease—bearing the burden with our loved ones throughout their long, dark years—must also find our way home as well, and for us it is also *the long way home.*

A Celebration of the Life of Edwin

*The following is the poem I wrote
for my husband's funeral.*

We've come to honour a man today
Who blessed our lives in many a way;
A loving father, a caring spouse,
Who loved to putter about the house.

And in the kitchen he did shine
With special meals at dinnertime;
From chili con carne (very tasty),
To stir fry, or an English pasty.

A very talented man was he
Whose main love was photography;
But into the picture went so much thought,
He'd take an age to snap the shot!

But the end results were worth the time;
And so he was a paradigm,
When his camera he would wield;
Outstanding in his special field.

He liked the other aspect too
Of standing in the camera's view;
And if a smile you would embrace,
Just stick a camera in his face!

With a sense of humour he was blessed
And made you laugh with many a jest;
His repartee was sharp and quick,
And he was also good at shtick.

His quick wit would make you laugh
And even if he pulled a gaffe,
He'd laugh at himself, along with you,
And that's what made him special too!

An elegant man, in English tweed,
Exuding casual comfort, indeed;
An English gentleman, through and through,
Kind, considerate, and good looking too!

But now he's gone to his heavenly home,
Where pain and sickness cannot roam;
He'll be happy there, so I must not cry,
Though now it's time to say goodbye.

* * *

Goodbye, Edwin. I love you!
~ *Marian Ritchie* ~